D1585838

CHURCHILL'S
POCKETBOOK OF
Primary Care Nursing

For Michael, Charlie and Alice and for my parents.

Churchill Livingstone:

Commissioning Editor: Ninette Premdas
Development Editor: Kim Benson
Production Manager: Yolanta Motylinska
Design/Production: Helius and Kneath Associates

CHURCHILL'S POCKETBOOK OF
Primary Care Nursing

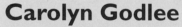
Anne Moger

Senior Lecturer, General Practice Nursing,
School of Health and Social Care,
Oxford Brookes University,
Oxford

Carolyn Godlee

General Practitioner
Summertown Health Centre,
Oxford

Simon Cartwright

General Practitioner
White Horse Medical Practice,
Faringdon, Oxfordshire

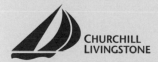

CHURCHILL
LIVINGSTONE

EDINBURGH LONDON NEW YORK OXFORD PHILADELPHIA
ST LOUIS SYDNEY TORONTO 2004

CHURCHILL LIVINGSTONE
An imprint of Elsevier Limited

First printed 2004

ISBN 0 443 10046 2

British Library Cataloguing in Publication Data
A catalogue record for this book is available from the British Library.

Library of Congress Cataloging in Publication Data
A catalog record for this book is available from the Library of Congress.

Note
Knowledge and best practice in this field are constantly changing. As new research and
experience broaden our knowledge, changes in practice, treatment and drug therapy
may become necessary or appropriate. Readers are advised to check the most current
information provided (i) on procedures featured or (ii) by the manufacturer of each
product to be administered, to verify the recommended dose or formula, the method and
duration of administration, and contraindications. It is the responsibility of the
practitioner, relying on their own experience and knowledge of the patient, to make
diagnoses, to determine dosages and the best treatment for each individual patient, and
to take all appropriate safety precautions. To the fullest extent of the law, neither the
publisher nor the editors assumes any liability for any injury and/or damage.

your source for books,
journals and multimedia
in the health sciences
www.elsevierhealth.com

The
publisher's
policy is to use
paper manufactured
from sustainable forests

Printed in China

CONTENTS

Foreword

Information for health professionals has never before been available in such abundance. Professional journals abound and the Internet and World Wide Web offer access to all kinds of materials. Most organisations have their own website for perusal, and every disease and condition is covered somewhere by someone offering expert advice and opinion.

Despite the proliferation of sources of information, nurses at the front line treating patients still need to be able to reach for a manual to give them instant access to relevant details about the illnesses they see on a day to day basis.

Today, nurses are frequently the patients' first point of contact with the health service. They work in a variety of settings, including GP surgeries, walk-in centres and minor injuries units. They assess, order tests, diagnose, refer, treat and may prescribe medicines. Each morning, such nurses are unlikely to know what problems will be presented by the patients to be seen in their clinic that day.

Nurses in primary care are also taking greater responsibility for chronic disease management and continuing care. This area of practice will continue to rise as the population ages. Already, 17.5 million people in the UK report having a chronic disease. Many of them, especially those over 65 years, have more than one condition, often compounded by the frailties of older age.

The new General Medical Services contract will reward primary healthcare teams for improving the quality of care for patients with chronic disease. It will be nurses who achieve much of this improvement in quality.

The breadth and range of symptoms and illnesses seen by nurses has grown exponentially, and each nurse needs to be confident in her ability to act independently and to know when to refer on to a doctor those whose needs fall outside her competence.

Nurses' knowledge must span less commonly seen conditions as well as the familiar, and they must be able to differentiate presenting symptoms from a range of possible options.

Modernising the NHS depends on increasing the capacity and capability of its nursing workforce. We need nurses to take on new roles and responsibilities to improve care and to generate more treatment options so that patients are offered real choice. At the same time, to protect standards, ensuring clinical practice is evidence or best practice based, is required of all professionals. Staying abreast of all that one needs to know is a challenge in itself.

Confidence grows with experience and increasing knowledge and competence, underpinned by education and training. It is also helped by having access to easy to use textbooks, kept close to hand to confirm or inform decisions about next steps.

The broad range of topics covered in this pocketbook, and the clear, concise information it contains, will render it a valuable source of help for all nurses in primary and community care.

Sarah Mullally
Chief Nursing Officer
Department of Health, England

Preface

This book was written as an adaptation to what has proved to be a popular and useful book primarily written for GPs. The wide professional readership indicated that it may prove even more valuable if it were expanded to include more detail in a variety of areas of primary care nursing expertise.

Nurses are increasingly finding themselves to be the first point of contact in primary care, particularly in rural areas away from large hospitals, and they need therefore to have expertise in areas such as the management of minor injuries. This has been dealt with in some detail in this edition, but is not intended to replace a comprehensive minor injuries manual. The aim is to provide a ready reference guide, when rapid access to practical information is required in order to support the decision-making process.

The treatment room section is aimed at nurses either new to or experienced in primary care. It provides some detailed information on commonly performed procedures that should prove useful to both practice nurses and their community nursing colleagues (district nurses, health visitors and school health nurses), particularly in relation to wound and leg ulcer management.

The sections on chronic disease management, which has become a priority within the new GMS Contract, have not been significantly adapted: they provide a comprehensive guide to management for all healthcare professionals in primary care.

Two symbols have been used to draw the reader's attention to important points:

 This denotes a useful tip, such as: 'The diagnosis of asthma in young children relies almost entirely on history.'

This indicates crucial information, such as: 'Call 999 and request ambulance paramedics as soon as MI is suspected, even if this is before the patient has been seen.'

We hope this book will support an increasingly multiprofessional approach to care for patients in primary care.

Abbreviations

A&E	accident and emergency	CT	computerised tomography
ABPI	ankle brachial pressure index	CVA	cerebrovascular accident
		CXR	chest X-ray
ACE	angiotensin converting enzyme		
		DEET	diethyltoluamide
ADH	antidiuretic hormone	DTP	diphtheria, tetanus, pertussis
AF	atrial fibrillation		
AFP	α-fetoprotein	DU	duodenal ulcer
AIDS	acquired immune deficiency syndrome	DVT	deep vein thrombosis
ALO	*Actinomyces*-like organisms	E/C	enteric coated
ASO	antistreptolysin O	ECG	electrocardiogram
AST	aspartate transaminase	EDD	estimated date of delivery
ASW	approved social worker	ELA	endometrial laser ablation
		ENT	ear, nose, throat
BCC	basal cell carcinoma	ERCP	endoscopic retrograde cholangiopancreaticogram
BCG	bacillus Calmette–Guèrin		
BMI	body mass index	ERPC	evacuation of retained products of conception
BNF	*British National Formulary*		
BP	blood pressure	ESR	erythrocyte sedimentation rate
BSI	British Standards Institution		
BTB	breakthrough bleeding	FBC	full blood count
		FOBs	faecal occult bloods
C&E	creatinine and electrolytes	FSH	follicle-stimulating hormone
CABG	coronary artery bypass graft		
CE	European Commission		
CHD	coronary heart disease	γ-GT	γ-glutamyl transferase
CMP	clinical management plan	GI	gastrointestinal
COC	combined oral contraceptive	GnRH	gonadotrophin-releasing hormone
COPD	chronic obstructive pulmonary disease	GORD	gastro-oesophageal reflux disease
CPR	cardiopulmonary resuscitation	GTN	glyceryl trinitrate
		GTT	glucose tolerance test
CRP	c-reactive protein	GU	gastric ulcer
CSF	cerebrospinal fluid	GUM	genitourinary medicine

HAV	hepatitis A virus	**MRSA**	methicillin resistant
Hb	haemoglobin		*Staphylococcus aureus*
HbA$_{1c}$	haemoglobin type A$_{1c}$	**MST**	morphine sulphate tablets
HCG	human chorionic gonadotrophin	**MSU**	mid-stream urine
HDL	high density lipoprotein	**NHSCSP**	NHS Cervical Screening Programme
HGV	heavy goods vehicle		
Hib	*Haemophilus influenza* B	**NICE**	National Institute of Clinical Excellence
HIV	human immunodeficiency virus	**NMC**	Nursing and Midwifery Council
HRT	hormone replacement therapy	**NPEF**	*Nurse Prescriber's Extended Formulary*
HVS	high vaginal swab	**NRT**	nicotine replacement therapy
IBS	irritable bowel syndrome	**NSAIDs**	non-steroidal anti-inflammatory drugs
IgA	immunoglobulin A		
IgM	immunoglobulin M	**OCD**	obsessive–compulsive disorder
IHD	ischaemic heart disease	**OTC**	over the counter
INR	international normalised ratio		
IUCD	intrauterine contraceptive device	**PE**	pulmonary embolus
IUS	intrauterine system	**PEFR**	peak expiratory flow rate
IVU	intravenous urogram	**PID**	pelvic inflammatory disease
		PMS	premenstrual syndrome
JVP	jugular venous pressure	**PMT**	premenstrual tension
		POP	progestogen-only pill
LFT	liver function tests	**POS**	polycystic ovarian syndrome
LH	luteinising hormone		
LMP	last menstrual period	**PPA**	Prescriptions Pricing Authority
LRTI	lower respiratory tract infection		
LVF	left ventricular failure	**PSA**	prostate-specific antigen
LVH	left ventricular hypertrophy	**PUO**	pyrexia of unknown origin
		PUVA	psoralens with UVA
MCH	mean corpuscular haemoglobin	**SC2**	self certificate
MCV	mean corpuscular volume	**SHBG**	sex-hormone binding globulin
MDI	metered-dose inhaler		
ME	myalagic encephalomyelitis	**SIDS**	sudden infant death syndrome
MI	myocardial infarct	**SLE**	systemic lupus erythematosus
MMR	measles, mumps, rubella		

SPF	sun protection factor		**U&E**	urea and electrolytes
S/R	slow release		**URTI**	upper respiratory tract infection
SSRI	selective serotonin reuptake inhibitor		**UTI**	urinary tract infection
STI	sexually transmitted infection		**UVA**	ultraviolet wavelength A
			UVB	ultraviolet wavelength B
TB	tuberculosis		**VA**	visual acuity
TCRE	transcervical resection of the endometrium		**VDRL**	venereal disease reference laboratory
TFTs	thyroid function tests			
TIA	transient ischaemic attack		**WHO**	World Health Organization
TOP	termination of pregnancy		**WSP**	white soft paraffin
TSH	thyroid stimulating hormone			

Dosage abbreviations

b.d.	twice daily		**PR**	per rectum
i.m.	intramuscular(ly)		**p.r.n.**	whenever required
i.v.	intravenous(ly)		**PV**	by the vaginal route
o.d.	(once) daily		**q.d.s.**	four times daily
o.m.	(once) every morning		**s.c.**	subcutaneous(ly)
o.n.	(once) every night		**stat.**	immediately
p.o.	by mouth		**t.d.s.**	three times daily

CONTRACEPTION

INTRODUCTION

The practice nurse with family planning training may play a significant role, e.g. diaphragm-fitting, pill-teaching and coil-checking.

Methods of contraception include: combined pills, progestogen-only pills, injectable and implanted progestogens, condoms, diaphragms, intrauterine contraceptive devices, natural methods and surgical sterilisation. Other methods, e.g. coitus interruptus, the use of spermicides alone and contraceptive sponges, are not discussed in this chapter, as their failure rates are relatively high.

Discussion of 'safe sex' and the prevention of HIV infection and other STIs should be part of the routine advice given to the sexually active. This is particularly important when counselling the very young. (Surveys suggest that about 50% of all under-16-year-old females have had intercourse.) 'Safe sex' means sex in which the exchange of bodily fluids is eliminated. 'Low-risk sex' means wet kissing, oral sex without ejaculation, and sexual intercourse using a condom. The use of the condom should be promoted in addition, often, to the main contraceptive. The advantages of fidelity within a sexual relationship, and, in the very young, of postponing intercourse, should be discussed in a non-judgemental way.

Always consider the possible STI risk when discussing contraception, particularly in the following situations:

- Young patient/early in sexual career.
- Emergency contraception request.
- IUCD request.
- TOP request.
- Assault.
- Patient symptomatic (pain, discharge, ulcers, intermenstrual bleeding, postcoital bleeding, breakthrough bleeding on COC, contact bleeding on taking cervical smear).
- Multiple partners or recent change of partner.
- Partner symptomatic.

GILLICK PRINCIPLES

A doctor must consider the following issues when the patient is under 16 years old:

- Whether the patient understands the potential risks and benefits of the treatment and the advice given.
- The value of parental support. Doctors must encourage young people to inform parents of the consultation and explore the reasons if the patient is unwilling to do so. The patient must be assured of confidentiality.

- Whether the patient is likely to have sexual intercourse without contraception.
- Whether the patient's physical or mental health is likely to suffer if he or she does not receive contraceptive advice or supplies.
- Whether the patient's best interests would require the provision of contraceptive advice or supplies, or both, without parental consent.

COMBINED ORAL CONTRACEPTIVE (COC)

STARTING THE COC

Assessment

History Ask about/think about possible contraindications.

Absolute contraindications
- DVT or emboli.
- Heart disease (valvular or ischaemic).
- Hypertension (>160/100).
- Hyperlipidaemia.
- Focal or severe migraine/TIAs.
- Cancer of the breast/cervix.
- From 4 weeks before to 2 weeks after major surgery.
- Rare:
  - liver disease (active)
  - polycythaemia; sickle cell anaemia
  - porphyria
  - hydatidiform mole (recent)
  - hyperprolactinaemia
  - diabetic complications.

Relative contraindications
- Family history of arterial disease.
- Diabetes.
- Hypertension (>160/95).
- Heavy cigarette smoking.
- Excessive weight.
- Age. (Smokers should stop the pill at the age of 35 years. There is no definite upper age limit in healthy non-smokers.)
- Common migraine.

Examination Check: ● weight ● blood pressure ● smear status.

Management
The following points should be considered and discussed, if appropriate:

Failure rate The failure rate is in the range 0.1–3/100 woman-years.

How to start the COC
- Start on day 1 or 2 and no extra contraceptive precautions are necessary.
- Alternatively, start on day 3–5 and take extra precautions for the first 7 days. (The COC may in fact be started on any day of the cycle, provided that extra precautions are taken for 7 days, but initial bleeding will be unpredictable.)

Ovulation The COC stops ovulation; 'periods' are light withdrawal bleeds.

Risks of taking the COC
- Smoking. Smoking >15 cigarettes per day increases the risk of circulatory disease by three times.
- Vascular disease in general is increased by about three times. (There is no statistically significant increased risk of myocardial infarction among pill users, unless they also smoke.)
- Hypertension develops in 5% of pill users after 5 years.
- There is a small increase in the risk of carcinoma of the breast during use and for 10 years after stopping the COC; this relative risk does not appear to be related to duration of use. It is more than counterbalanced by the protective effect against cancers of the ovary and endometrium.

Side-effects
- Breakthrough bleeding. (This usually settles within 2–3 months.)
- Nausea, breast tenderness, weight gain, PMT, bloating (fluid retention), depression, vaginal discharge (secondary to cervical erosion), headaches, reduced libido, chloasma.

Gastrointestinal upset Vomiting and severe diarrhoea lead to reduced hormone absorption. Take extra contraceptive precautions for the period of illness and for 7 days afterwards.

What to do if a pill is missed

The most risky pills to miss are those in the first or last week of the pack, as the 7-day hormone gap is lengthened. If a pill is missed, take the missed pill at once and take the next pill at the usual time. If missed for less than 12 hours assume no loss of contraception. If missed for more than 12 hours take extra contraceptive precautions for 7 days. If more than one pill is missed, take two pills at once (if on a phased pill, the most recent two pills of those missed) and take the next pill at the usual time. Take extra contraceptive precautions for 7 days. If there are less than seven pills left in the packet, avoid lengthening the 7-day hormone gap by starting the next pack without a break.

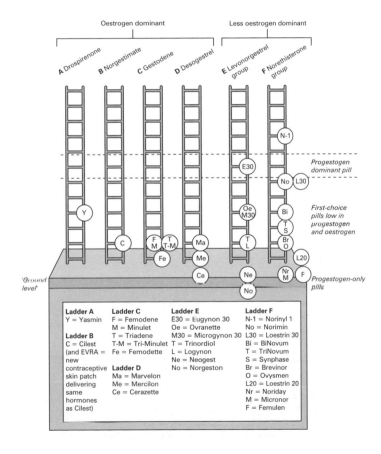

Reproduced with permission from Guillebaud J 2004 Contraception: your questions answered, 4th edn. Churchill Livingstone, Edinburgh

Prescribing Ideally, use the lowest strength of pill that does not cause breakthrough bleeding (BTB) The dose of oestrogen (ethinyloestradiol) should normally be no more than 20–35 μg. With any chosen progestogen there should be a preference for the lowest acceptable dose (i.e. not so low as to cause BTB).

Pills containing the third-generation progestogens (desogestrel or gestodene), e.g. Femodene, Marvelon, Mercilon, Minulet, Triadene and Tri-Minulet, increase the risk of DVT. In 100,000 women, the approximate number developing a DVT in 1 year is:

- for women taking one of these six pills, 25
- for women taking one of the other COCs, 15
- for women who are pregnant, 60
- for other healthy women, 5.

Women with risk factors for venous disease (including women with a BMI > 30, those with marked varicose veins, those with an immobility problem and those with a family history of DVT) should not use these pills.

Common choices for women free of risk factors for arterial disease under the age of 30 years are pills delivering levonorgestrel or norethisterone, e.g. Microgynon 30, Loestrin 20 or 30, or Ovran 30. Women with risk factors for arterial disease or those who are relatively intolerant of pills containing levonorgestrel or norethisterone may do better on a pill containing a third-generation progestogen.

Most patients seem to do better on a monophasic pill than on a triphasic one in the first instance.

Drug interactions
Liver enzyme inducers, e.g. phenytoin, carbamazepine, griseofulvin and phenobarbitone, increase the metabolism, and thus elimination in the bile, of both oestrogen and progestogen. If the patient is on a liver enzyme inducer, start a higher dose pill (≥50 μg oestrogen). Consider 'tricycling' (i.e. taking 3 or 4 packets of monophasic tablets without a break followed by a short tablet-free interval of 4 days).

> Certain broad-spectrum antibiotics (e.g. ampicillin, tetracyclines and griseofulvin) alter gut flora and reduce oestrogen absorption. Take extra precautions for the duration of treatment and for 7 days afterwards. Long-term treatment with antibiotics does not require extra precautions, as resistant flora develop.

Follow-up The first follow-up is at 3 months. Subsequent follow-ups are at 6–12-month intervals.

Check: • new risk factors • smoking status • weight change • BP • smear status.

Management of subsequent problems

Breakthrough bleeding
- Ask about COC compliance or vomiting (prevents COC absorption).
- Liver enzyme inducing drugs (e.g. phenytoin) can cause BTB.
- Consider pregnancy.
- Check for cervical lesions if BTB is persistent.
- (*Chlamydia* may cause a blood-stained discharge.)

If BTB persists for >2–3 months after starting the COC try an equivalent pill with a different progestogen (see pill ladder, p. 5) or a pill with a higher oestrogen or progestogen content or change to a triphasic pill.

Absent withdrawal bleed Absent withdrawal bleeds are harmless in themselves. Consider pregnancy. Consider changing to a pill with a lower dose of progestogen.

Side-effects As a general rule, for all minor side-effects, reduce the dose where possible (this usually means reducing the dose of the progestogen, as nearly all pill-takers are on 30–35 µg of the oestrogen), or change to a pill containing a different progestogen.

The following side-effects are due to a relative oestrogen excess, and may be alleviated by changing to a progestogen-dominant pill (e.g. Loestrin 30 or Eugynon 30): • nausea • dizziness • PMT • cyclical weight gain • 'bloating' • vaginal discharge.

The following side-effects are due to a relative progestogen excess, and may be alleviated by changing to an oestrogen-dominant pill (e.g. Mercilon, Trinordiol, Logynon, Marvelon or Cilest): • vaginal dryness • sustained weight gain • depression • loss of libido • lassitude • breast tenderness • acne • hirsutism.

Changing from one pill to another If the new pill has the same oestrogen dose or higher than the old pill, start it after a 7-day gap. If the new pill has a lower oestrogen dose than the old pill, start it immediately after the previous pack without a break.

To postpone a period (e.g. for a holiday) Start the next pack immediately, without a break. (With phased pills, except Synphase, take the extra pills from the last phase of the new pack. This will postpone the period by the same number of days as there are tablets in the last phase of the pack.)

Stopping the pill to conceive Ideally, use an alternative method of contraception for 3 months and until one natural period has passed. Preconceptual counselling is important (see p. 22).

PROGESTOGEN-ONLY PILL (POP)

The POP is particularly useful for the following:

- Older women – especially those over 35 years old who smoke. (In women over 40 years old the POP is as effective as the COC.) It can relieve PMT and climacteric symptoms.
- Lactating women.
- Women in whom the COC is contraindicated by e.g. hypertension, diabetes, migraine, thrombosis and embolus.
- Women with troublesome oestrogenic side-effects from the COC, e.g. fluid retention, cyclical weight gain, headache and chloasma.
- Women awaiting major surgery.

STARTING THE POP

Assessment

History Ask about/think about possible contraindications.

Contraindications
- Past or present severe arterial disease, or an exceptionally high risk of the same.
- Recent hydatidiform mole.
- Porphyria.

 There is no evidence of an increased risk of thrombosis.

Examination Check: • weight • blood pressure • smear status.

Management
The following points should be considered and discussed:

Failure rate The overall failure rate is in the range 0.3–4/100 woman-years.

Irregular bleeding or amenorrhoea These may occur. Most women have a cycle of between 25 and 35 days. The blood loss is light.

Drug interactions Efficacy is reduced by enzyme-inducing drugs.

 Antibiotics do not affect the POP.

How to start the POP
- Start on day 1 (the first day of the period) and no extra contraceptive precautions are necessary.
- If starting in mid-cycle, take extra precautions for the first 7 days.
- If changing from a COC, start the POP immediately, without a 7-day gap. No extra precautions are necessary.
- Take the POP regularly every day (no breaks) at the same time, within 2–3 hours. It is maximally effective 5 hours after taking it. If a couple normally have intercourse in the morning, the POP should ideally be taken in the evening.

What to do if a pill is missed
Take it as soon as it is remembered and carry on with the next pill at the right time. If a pill is taken more than 3 hours late, protection may be lost. Continue normal pill-taking and take extra contraceptive precautions for 7 days. Emergency (oral or IUCD) postcoital contraception (see p. 10) should be offered after any unprotected intercourse which occurs during the 7 days after missing one pill by more than 3 hours.

Complications There is an increased incidence of ectopic pregnancies.

Side-effects Breakthrough bleeding, nausea and breast tenderness usually settle after 2–3 months.

Vomiting and severe diarrhoea In the event of these symptoms, continue normal pill-taking and take extra precautions for the period of illness and for 7 days afterwards.

Follow-up The first follow-up is at 3 months. Subsequent follow-ups are at 6–12 month intervals.
    Check: • new risk factors • weight change • BP • smear status.

INJECTABLE PROGESTOGENS

Injectable progestogens inhibit ovulation. The failure rate is 0–2/100 woman-years. The contraindications are as for the POP. They are especially useful for forgetful pill-takers in whom other methods may be inappropriate or contraindicated. The main disadvantage is that the method is irreversible for at least 3 months, and early side-effects may therefore have to be tolerated for this length of time.
    The main side-effects are: • breakthrough bleeding • amenorrhoea with delay in return to fertility for up to 1 year • weight gain.
    The usual treatment is 150 mg Depo-Provera i.m. 3-monthly. The first

injection should be given within the first 5 days of the cycle to give immediate contraceptive effect.

It is important for the nurse admistering the injection to ascertain that it is not being given late. With Depo provera, there is a 3-day period of leeway beyond the recommended 13 weeks. After this time, emergency contraception needs to be considered.

PROGESTOGEN-RELEASING IMPLANT (IMPLANON)

This etonogestrel-releasing single flexible rod is inserted subdermally into the lower surface of the upper arm.

- It should be inserted during the first 5 days of the cycle to give immediate contraceptive effect.
- It is effective for up to 3 years. In women with a BMI >35 it should be replaced after 2 years.
- The contraindications are as for the POP.
- The contraceptive effect is immediately reversible on removal of the implant.

POSTCOITAL (EMERGENCY) CONTRACEPTION

Postcoital contraception is sometimes needed as an emergency measure to prevent pregnancy when unprotected intercourse has put the woman at risk.

HORMONAL EMERGENCY CONTRACEPTION

Assessment

History Ask about:
- contraindications:
  - pregnancy
  - porphyria
- LMP
- normal menstrual cycle
- times of all unprotected intercourse during the present cycle
- present method of contraception.

Hormonal postcoital contraception should be considered if a woman has unprotected intercourse in the 7 days after the following situations.

- In a COC taker:
  - if the pill-free interval has been lengthened to 9 days or more
  - more than one pill has been missed in the first 7 days of the packet
  - more than three pills have been missed in the middle 7 days of the packet
  - more than one pill has been missed in the last 7 days of the packet, and the next packet is not run straight on
  - several pills have been missed throughout the packet.
- In a POP taker: if a pill is taken more than 3 hours late.

Management

Advice
- The failure rate is 1–2%.
- The sooner it is started after unprotected intercourse, the greater the efficacy.
- Nausea occurs occasionally. If vomiting occurs within 2 hours of taking either dose, a further dose should be taken together with an anti-emetic.
- The next period may be early or late.
- Barrier methods should be used until the next period.
- Discuss future contraception.
- There is no known teratogenic effect if the method fails.
- A pill taker should continue to take her usual pills in the normal way and be warned that she may get spotting in that cycle.
- Double the dose of levonorgestrel if the woman is taking enzyme-inducing drugs. There is no need to increase the dose if on broad-spectrum antibiotics.
- This method may be used more than once in any one cycle.

Prescribing Levonorgestrel 1.5 mg (2 tablets) as a single dose as soon as possible after coitus (preferably within 12 hours, but no later than after 72 hours). Also available OTC.

> Hormonal postcoital contraception is effective for up to 72 hours after intercourse, in preventing implantation.

Follow-up This is not usually necessary. It may be arranged 1 month later in order to establish that the patient is not pregnant. Discuss future contraception.

EMERGENCY IUCD

Assessment

History Ask about:
- Contraindications. The majority of general contraindications to the IUCD apply (see p. 14). However, the IUCD *can* be used for postcoital

contraception in women with a past history of an ectopic pregnancy, in nulliparous women and in women with a recent history of pelvic inflammatory disease (providing antibiotic cover is given).
- LMP.
- Normal menstrual cycle.
- Times of all unprotected intercourse during the present cycle.
- Present method of contraception.

Management

Advice
- The IUCD can be fitted up to 5 days after unprotected intercourse or up to 5 days after the most probable calculated date of ovulation, e.g. day 19 of a regular 28-day cycle.
- It can be removed after the next period or kept for long-term contraception, if appropriate.

CONDOM

The failure rate of the condom is <1/100 couple-years if used correctly.

Management

Every opportunity should be taken for the nurse to give advice about the benefits of safe sex. Suitable opportunities would be:

- The travel health consultation (see p. 211).
- The well-man health check.
- The new patient registration medical.

> It is essential when giving advice about the use of condoms that their value in the prevention of sexually transmitted infection is stressed as well as their benefits as a contraceptive method.

Advice
- A condom should be used every time intercourse takes place.
- Use a new condom each time you have sex.
- Check the 'use by' date on the packet and look for the BSI Kitemark and the European CE mark.
- Take care removing the condom from the packet as sharp finger nails or rings can damage the condom.
- Find the teat or closed end of the condom and squeeze to expel air; this will make it easier to roll the condom on the right way round.

- Put the condom on when the penis is fully erect and before it touches the vagina or genital area.
- Still holding the end, roll the condom all the way down to the base of the penis.
- If it will not go all the way down, it is probably inside out. Start again using a new condom, in case there is already sperm on the first one.
- After ejaculation and before the erection is lost, hold the condom in place while pulling out slowly to avoid spilling any of the sperm.
- Take off the condom, wrap it and put it in a bin, not down the toilet.
- Lubricants may be used with condoms, but remember never to use condoms with oil-based products such as body oils, sun cream or petroleum jelly, as these can damage the condom and make it more likely to split.
- If the condom fails for any reason during intercourse, emergency contaception may be required, so visit the doctor, nurse or family planning clinic as soon as possible for advice.
- The condom should always be used with a spermicide.

 The condom is the only contraceptive which effectively protects against STI and AIDS.

Administration
- The condom is not prescribable on FP10 (GP10 in Scotland), but is free at Family Planning Clinics and most GP surgeries. Available OTC.

DIAPHRAGM

The failure rate of the diaphragm is about 4/100 woman-years.

At the initial fitting, check the smear status. Advise the woman to practise insertion at home and, if appropriate, to use the diaphragm during intercourse with additional contraception until the first follow-up.

Management

Advice
- Always use a spermicide with the diaphragm.
- Insert the diaphragm any time prior to intercourse.
- Insert additional spermicide (a pessary or foam) prior to each episode of intercourse taking place more than 2 hours after initial insertion.
- Leave the diaphragm in place for at least 6 hours after intercourse, up to a maximum of 24 hours.
- Check the diaphragm intermittently for holes.
- A diaphragm usually lasts for 1–2 years.

Follow-up
- This should be about 10 days or shortly after fitting, and then annually.
- Check the position of the diaphragm, after the woman has inserted it herself.
- Recheck:
  - if the woman's weight changes by more than 3.5 kg (8 lb)
  - at the 6-week postnatal check
  - after vaginal surgery.

Administration
- Prescribe the device and a spermicide on FP10 (GP10 in Scotland). The cost and administration of the diaphragm can be claimed from the PPA.

INTRAUTERINE CONTRACEPTIVE DEVICE (IUCD)

The failure rate of the IUCD is in the range 0.3–2/100 woman-years. It renders the endometrium unsuitable for implantation.

Assessment

History Ask about/think about contraindications:
- undiagnosed irregular genital tract bleeding
- pregnancy
- pelvic inflammatory disease (within the previous 6 months)
- previous ectopic pregnancy
- distortion of the uterine cavity
- past history of bacterial endocarditis or valve replacement
- the IUCD is less suitable for nulliparous women and those with menorrhagia or dysmenorrhoea (see IUS, p. 16).

Management

Insertion Insertion should be in the first 14 days of the cycle and the contraceptive effect is immediate.

Women at high risk of chlamydial infection should be screened (see p. 46). Take swabs for *Chlamydia* and await results before inserting the IUCD. Those at high risk include (see also p. 2):

- age <25 years
- more than one sexual partner in the preceding 12 months
- emergency contraception request
- previous STI
- symptoms of infection.

Advice
- The patient should check the threads weekly for 6 weeks, and monthly thereafter, ideally right at the end of a period.
- Warn the patient about crampy pains for 2–3 days after insertion.
- Tampons can be used.
- Irregular spotting may occur in the first cycle.
- Periods may be heavier and more prolonged.
- Any normal discharge may be heavier.
- Menstrual irregularity and pelvic pain require exclusion of an ectopic pregnancy.

Follow-up At 6 weeks, and then annually:
- Check threads.
- Check smear status.
- Exclude anaemia, if appropriate.
- Consider replacement/alternative contraception, if appropriate.

Main disadvantages of IUCDs
- Dysmenorrhoea and menorrhagia (especially in the first 3 months).
- Pelvic infection (see p. 45).
- Perforation.
- Expulsion.
- Lost threads. If the threads are lost, exclude pregnancy and advise temporary alternative contraception. The device may be within the uterus, have perforated the uterus or have been expelled. Try retrieving the threads by inserting Spencer–Wells forceps into the endocervical canal. If unsuccessful, arrange an ultrasound. If the IUCD is seen to be in the uterine cavity and does not need changing, leave in situ. Arrange gynaecological assessment, if appropriate.
- Intrauterine pregnancy. If the IUCD is in situ, there is an increased risk of miscarriage and, therefore, of infection. The risk can be reduced if the IUCD is gently removed as early as possible. If the pregnancy is >12 weeks, refer to an obstetrician.
- Ectopic pregnancy. (1 in 10–20 pregnancies occurring with the IUCD are extrauterine.) The patient should be advised to report pelvic pain or abnormal bleeding.

Removal All IUCDs are licensed for 5 years use. They should be removed during a period or following 7 days abstinence or protected intercourse. If an IUCD is fitted in a woman over the age of 40, it may remain in the uterus until the menopause.

   If the woman is planning a pregnancy, she should delay conception until 1 month after removal of the IUCD, to allow time for normal endometrium to regenerate.

   The IUCD should be removed 2 years after the menopause in women under the age of 50 years, and 1 year after the menopause in women over the age of 50 years.

> If the IUCD is removed intermenstrually, alternative contraception should be used for 7 days prior to removal.

Administration
- Prescribe the device on form FP10 (GP10 stock order form in Scotland).
- Claim for insertion and claim for the cost and administration of the IUCD from the PPA on form FP10 (GP10 stock order form in Scotland).

INTRAUTERINE PROGESTOGEN-ONLY SYSTEM (MIRENA/IUS)

This is highly effective, with a failure rate of 0.2/100 woman-years. It results in a lower ectopic pregnancy rate than in women using no method. It usually leads to oligomenorrhoea or amenorrhoea, and is therefore suitable for women with heavy periods. Dysmenorrhoea and the risk of pelvic infection are reduced, compared to normal, and it is therefore suitable for nulliparous women. It is effective for 5 years. Return of fertility is rapid after removal. Fitting should be in the first 14 days of the cycle. If fitted after day 7 of the cycle, condoms should be used for the following 7 days.

Insertion is more painful than with standard IUCDs in view of an inserter of greater diameter, and intermenstrual spotting is a common problem in the early months of use. Spotting may occasionally continue for up to 6 months.

NATURAL BIRTH CONTROL

CALENDAR METHOD

This should only be considered when periods are regular. The period of abstinence required is often long. In a 28-day cycle, ovulation is around day 14 and the fertile period is between days 8 and 17. The released ovum survives for 1 day. The sperm survives for up to 6 days within the female body.

Method of calculation
- Define the shortest and longest menstrual cycle over the previous 12 months.

- To derive the first day of the fertile period, subtract 20 from the length of the shortest cycle. (14 days = maximum length of a luteal phase; 6 days = maximum sperm survival.)
- To derive the last day of the fertile period, subtract 11 from the length of the longest cycle. (12 days = minimum length of a luteal phase; 1 day = maximum ovum survival.)

This method has a high failure rate, even with good compliance.

PERSONA

This machine is available over the counter. The woman's hormone profile is analysed using daily urine testing strips, giving an indication of the 'safe period'.

MUCOTHERMAL METHOD

Intercourse should be confined to between 72 hours following the detection of ovulation and the onset of the next menstrual period. Ovulation can be detected by:

- a rise in basal body temperature
- thinning of cervical mucus (Billing's method).

STERILISATION

Both partners must accept that surgical sterilisation should be considered to be irreversible. Sterilisation should not be performed immediately postpartum or post-TOP, as regret is more likely if the decision is made at a time of stress.

The failure rate of sterilisation is about 0.2/100 woman-years.

Assessment

History Ask about: • the age of the man and the woman • the number and ages of their children, and their health • the menstrual history • present contraception • relationship stability.

Discuss:

- the irreversibility of sterilisation
- alternative forms of contraception
- the pros and cons of male versus female sterilisation
- complications (these should be discussed by the surgeon).

Laparoscopic sterilisation is usually performed as a day case under general or local anaesthetic. It may require 1 week off work.

Vasectomy is usually a local anaesthetic outpatient procedure. Sperm clearance takes about 20 ejaculations. It takes two sterile semen specimens, 4 months after vasectomy, 2 weeks apart, to confirm its contraceptive effect.

Examination Examine the male genitalia for vasectomy.

Administration
The patient should sign a consent form, as appropriate.

HORMONAL CONTRACEPTION IN THE PERIMENOPAUSE

Contraception should be continued for 1 year after the LMP in women over the age of 50 years, and for 2 years in women under the age of 50. If any potentially fertile woman requires HRT, non-hormonal contraception is necessary.

THE COC
Women who smoke and those with other cardiovascular risk factors should stop the COC at the age of about 35. Fit, normotensive non-smokers with no family history of cardiovascular disease may continue the COC until the age of 50 (consider a 20 µg oestrogen pill, as the absolute risk of cardiovascular disease and breast cancer increases with age).

Synthetic oestrogens in the COC reduce perimenopausal symptoms, but they do not protect against osteoporosis or cardiovascular disease as do natural oestrogens in HRT.

THE POP
The POP does not usually disguise the menopause. Vasomotor symptoms may occur while taking it and the serum FSH may be raised. The failure rate in older women is minimal and is equivalent to the COC in younger women.

In order to establish whether or not natural periods have ceased, stop the COC/POP, and use non-hormonal contraception:

- The onset of vasomotor symptoms together with amenorrhoea indicates the menopause, and contraception only needs to be continued for 1 year.
- If periods return the COC/POP may be resumed. (Whether amenorrhoea occurs or periods return, HRT may be started with non-hormonal contraception, if appropriate.)
- Two FSH levels of >30 IU/l, 3 months apart, indicate the menopause.

POSTPARTUM CONTRACEPTION

No contraception is necessary for the first 25 days postpartum. If breast-feeding, avoid the COC, as oestrogen may inhibit lactation.

When to start

- COC and POP: can be started at 21 days postpartum.
- IUCD: can be inserted at 6 weeks (postnatal check) or at 12 weeks after a Caesarian section.
- Diaphragm: can be fitted at 6 weeks (postnatal check).

OBSTETRICS

PRECONCEPTUAL COUNSELLING

Preconceptual counselling ensures that the woman is fully informed about measures which may be taken to protect herself and the developing foetus during any future pregnancy.

Assessment

History Ask about: • past medical and obstetric history, family history and social problems • present contraception.

Examination
- Check the pre-pregnancy blood pressure.
- Perform a cervical smear, if due.

Investigations
- Rubella antibodies should be checked before the first pregnancy. If the woman is non-immune she should be vaccinated and should avoid conception for 1 month.
- If the woman has had a previous large baby (>4.5 kg), consider performing a fasting blood glucose and a modified GTT.
- Arrange haemoglobin electrophoresis to exclude thalassaemia trait in those from southern Europe, the Indian subcontinent and the Far East, and sickle cell trait in Afro-Caribbeans. Refer couples who are both heterozygous.

Management

Advice

Smoking and alcohol Women should be advised to stop smoking and to reduce their alcohol intake to a minimum.

Diet and nutrition
- Advise a well-balanced diet.
- Advise a diet rich in folic acid (green vegetables, bread, potatoes, fruit and fortified cereals). Advise all women to take supplements of folic acid, 400 µg per day, from before conception to 12 weeks of gestation. This reduces the risk of neural tube defects. (Folic acid can be prescribed on FP10 (GP10 in Scotland) or bought OTC.)
- To minimise the risk of listeriosis, avoid unpasteurised soft cheeses, cooked chilled foods, prepacked salads and pâtés.
- To minimise the risk of toxoplasmosis, avoid undercooked meat, wash all vegetables and fruit prior to consumption, and avoid handling soil or cat faeces.
- Avoid high vitamin A intake.
- Avoid peanuts.

- Consider a high-calcium diet or calcium supplements for women at high risk, e.g. grand multiparous women or those who are socially deprived.

Contraception If oral contraception or an IUCD is being used, one natural period without contraception should ideally be allowed before conception.

Referral

Obstetric problems
- Previous miscarriages: if the woman has had three or more miscarriages, refer for assessment of, e.g. cervical incompetence (which tends to cause mid-trimester miscarriages) or chromosomal abnormalities.
- Previous still births, foetal abnormalities or a family history of foetal abnormalities: refer for genetic counselling where this is likely to be beneficial. Advise, where appropriate, on antenatal screening and diagnosis. If the patient has a previous history or family history of a neural tube defect, advise her to take folic acid 5 mg daily from 1 month prior to stopping contraception to 12 weeks of gestation.

Medical problems
- Hypertension: refer for assessment. Methyldopa and some beta blockers, e.g. propranolol, are known to be safe and effective in pregnancy.
- Diabetes: refer for assessment. Perinatal mortality is around 10%, even with excellent control of blood sugar, which is crucial. The incidence of congenital abnormalities can be significantly reduced by good blood sugar control both before and during pregnancy. HbA_{1c} levels should be checked before stopping contraception.
- Epilepsy: refer for assessment. Congenital abnormalities are more than twice as common as usual. All anticonvulsants increase the incidence of foetal abnormalities to varying degrees, and this has to be assessed against the risk of untreated epilepsy and convulsions during pregnancy.

BOOKING VISIT

The booking visit is ideally between 8 and 14 weeks, and usually requires a 20–30 minute appointment.

Diagnosis
Pregnancy can be confirmed by home or laboratory testing of an early morning urine specimen taken after a missed period, measuring urinary HCG.

 A diagnosis of pregnancy can usually be made on the history alone.

History Ask about:
- LMP (and degree of certainty of that date), and calculate EDD
- age, occupation, race of both patient and partner (if appropriate), medical and obstetric problems (see p. 23), socioeconomic background, family history, alcohol, smoking and dental hygiene.

Examination • Height • weight • heart • lungs • legs (for varicose veins) • abdomen.
 Vaginal examination is unnecessary.

Investigations
- Urine: check for protein and sugar and send an MSU.
- Bloods:
  - Hb
  - ABO and rhesus groups and antibodies
  - VDRL and hepatitis B status
  - HIV status (this is now routinely checked with patient consent)
  - rubella antibodies
  - consider testing for haemoglobinopathies (see p. 22)
  - arrange serum AFP and a 'triple test'/integrated test if required at appropriate times (see p. 26).
- Ultrasound scan (see p. 25): consider
  - a dating scan at 7–11 weeks
  - a nuchal scan at 10–13 weeks
  - an anomaly scan at 18–20 weeks.

Management
After assessing risk factors, discuss the most appropriate form of antenatal and intrapartum care. The usual options are 'shared care' (the patient's care is shared between hospital doctors and GPs, and the mother is delivered by the hospital team), community care (involving the GP and the community midwives) and home delivery. Arrangements and criteria for low-risk community units will vary according to the locality. Refer as appropriate.

Advice
- Discuss diet (see p. 22).
- Discuss prenatal screening and diagnosis (see p. 25), as appropriate.
- Discuss the woman's concerns and expectations with regard to the pregnancy and delivery.

SUBSEQUENT ANTENATAL VISITS

Follow-up intervals vary. Normal multigravidae require at least six antenatal check-ups at 12, 16, 22, 30, 36 and 40 weeks. In addition, normal primigravidae require check-ups at 26, 34, 38 and 41 weeks. In practice, most pregnant women tend to be reviewed 4-weekly until 28 weeks, 2-weekly until 36 weeks and weekly thereafter.

Diagnosis

History Ask about: • general health • gestation.

Examination
- Blood pressure.
- Look for oedema.
- Fundal height and foetal presentation (from 32 weeks).
- Foetal movements/foetal heart (Doppler, e.g. Sonicaid, can detect the foetal heart from 12 weeks of gestation).

Investigations
- Urinalysis for protein and sugar.
- At 28 and 36 weeks re-check Hb and ABO and rhesus groups.
- Prenatal screening (see below), as appropriate.

Administration
Complete form Mat B1 at 26 weeks, if appropriate.

PRENATAL SCREENING AND DIAGNOSIS

SCREENING TESTS

All women may be offered ultrasound, serum AFP and the triple test or integrated test as part of routine screening. Discussion of the pros and cons of these tests must take account of the patient's feelings regarding termination of pregnancy. False-positive results can cause considerable unnecessary anxiety. Diagnostic tests are necessary to confirm a postive screening test.

Ultrasound
- Dating scans: estimation of gestation is more accurate early in pregnancy, from 7–11 weeks. Helpful if the LMP is uncertain.
- Nuchal scans: performed at 10–13 weeks can detect 80% of Down's syndrome babies (only available privately in some areas).
- Foetal anomaly scans: best performed at 18–20 weeks and usually organised routinely. Various abnormalities can be detected, including:
  - cranial and neural tube defects
  - abnormalities of the heart, chest and abdominal organs
  - cleft lip and palate.

Serum AFP This is performed from 15 weeks. A high level indicates a higher risk of neural tube defect, or twins. A low level indicates a higher risk of Down's syndrome.

Triple test This is a blood test, performed between 15 and 21 weeks and in some areas only available privately; it estimates the risk of Down's syndrome and neural tube defects. The estimated risk of Down's syndrome is based on serum AFP, HCG and unconjugated oestriol, as well as maternal age. The risk of a neural tube defect is based on AFP alone. It is particularly helpful for older mothers. (The risk of Down's at age 35 years is 1:400, while at age 40 it is 1:100.) Several versions of the same test are available from different centres, e.g. St. Bartholomew's Hospital, London, Leeds, Cambridge and Kettering.

Integrated test This test combines a 10–13 week nuchal scan and blood test for pregnancy-associated plasma protein, together with a 15–21 week blood test for AFP, HCG, unconjugated oestriol and inhibin-A. The measurements are integrated into a single screening result, taking account of maternal age. The test detects 90% of Down's syndrome babies and 80% of spina bifida babies. Other tests involving a nuchal scan and blood tests are also available. In most areas they are only available privately.

DIAGNOSTIC TESTS

Chorionic villus biopsy This is performed at 8–12 weeks, allowing termination in the first trimester if an abnormality is confirmed. It enables early detection of chromosomal abnormalities and other rare genetic diseases. There is a 1–2% miscarriage rate. Limb deformities are a rare risk of this biopsy.

Amniocentesis This is performed at 15–16 weeks, allowing termination before 20 weeks if an abnormality is confirmed. The miscarriage rate is 0.5–1%. It detects Down's syndrome, X-linked disorders (e.g. haemophilia and Duchenne muscular dystrophy) and some inborn errors of metabolism (e.g. Tay–Sachs disease). Results of fluid analysis for AFP usually take 1 week, while cell culture for karyotype or biochemistry takes 3 weeks. Anti-D is given if the woman is rhesus negative.

BLEEDING IN EARLY PREGNANCY (<14 weeks)

Diagnosis

History Ask about:
- the extent of the bleeding, including the presence of clots, and whether or not pelvic pain is present
- rhesus blood group.

Examination Perform a vaginal examination in order to establish whether the cervix is open or closed. This is not necessary if the bleeding is slight and there is no pain. An open cervix suggests an inevitable abortion and a non-viable pregnancy. Alternatively, an urgent ultrasound scan can assess viability, avoiding the need for a vaginal examination.

Management
For vaginal spotting without pain:

- Telephone advice is usually adequate.
- Advise to rest at home.

For vaginal bleeding with pain:

- Mild discomfort and light bleeding can usually be managed at home.
- Worsening pain usually suggests the need for admission, especially if it is associated with the passing of clots.
- An open cervix confirms the need for admission. If the bleeding is heavy, remove any products of conception, with a gloved hand, and give syntometrine i.m., 1 ml.

> Vaginal bleeding at >12 weeks in a rhesus-negative woman requires an injection of anti-D 500 IU i.m. within 72 hours of the start of bleeding. At <12 weeks, anti-D only needs to be given if the bleeding is heavy, e.g. ERPC is required.

If the miscarriage is complete (i.e. products have been passed and the pain and bleeding have settled):

- Advise rest at home and arrange early review.
- Tell the patient to contact the doctor if bleeding recurs.
- Give an explanation, as appropriate:
  - the likely cause is foetal abnormality or implantation failure
  - investigation is not useful in first-trimester miscarriages unless there have been three or more.
- Bereavement counselling is often important.

If the pregnancy continues and the symptoms settle:

- Review and consider arranging a scan to exclude a missed abortion.
- Explain that bleeding in pregnancy does not increase the risk of foetal abnormalities.

Administration
Complete form GMS2 (GPM maternity claim form in Scotland).

Criteria
- A patient miscarrying after the 8th week attracts a fee.
- A patient miscarrying before the 8th week must already be registered for maternity care, otherwise no fee is payable.
- Therapeutic abortions do not qualify for maternity fees.

BLEEDING IN LATER PREGNANCY

After 14 weeks, admission should be arranged when bleeding occurs, with or without pain. Bleeding with severe pain is likely to be due to placental abruption. If the woman's blood group is rhesus negative she requires an injection of anti-D 500 IU i.m. within 72 hours of the start of bleeding.

 Do not perform a vaginal examination after 14 weeks in case of placenta praevia.

NAUSEA AND VOMITING

Vomiting in pregnancy can be extremely debilitating and the patient often requires considerable support and reassurance.

Management
- Explain that the symptoms are likely to resolve by 14–16 weeks.
- Encourage fluids (carbonated drinks can be helpful) and frequent, small, plain meals.
- Consider drug treatment if the symptoms are severe, e.g. promethazine 25 mg mane, 50 mg nocte.
- Consider admission if vomiting is prolonged or dehydration is a concern.

HEARTBURN

Heartburn usually worsens as pregnancy progresses. It can be exacerbated by oral iron.

Management
- Recommend frequent small meals.
- Prescribe an antacid with a low sodium content, e.g. Maalox 10 ml after meals or p.r.n.

SWOLLEN ANKLES

Swollen ankles are common in pregnancy.

Management
- Exclude pre-eclampsia. (Check for more generalised oedema, hypertension and/or proteinuria.)
- Advise the patient to avoid long periods of standing. If oedema becomes uncomfortable, advise her to sit with the ankles above the level of the hips when possible, and to wear support stockings or tights (see below).

VARICOSE VEINS

Varicose veins tend to worsen with each pregnancy.

Management
- Avoid long periods of standing.
- Advise the patient to sit with the ankles above the level of the hips when resting, and to wear support stockings or tights. Support stockings are obtainable on FP10 (GP10 in Scotland) in three grades. Support tights are usually more comfortable, but are only available OTC. Support hosiery should ideally be put on before getting out of bed in the morning.
- Surgery should be avoided until the woman has completed her family.

GLYCOSURIA

Misleading detection of postprandial glycosuria can be avoided by testing an early morning specimen.

Modified glucose tolerance test
After two episodes of glycosuria a modified glucose tolerance test should be performed:

- Measure fasting blood glucose.
- Give a 75 g oral load of glucose (e.g. 350 ml of Lucozade).
- Measure blood glucose again after 2 hours.

Management

Fasting values of >5.8 mmol/l or 2-hour values of >7.8 mmol/l suggest gestational diabetes, and the patient should be referred urgently.

PROTEINURIA

A trace of protein in the urine can be ignored.

Management

- Check the blood pressure to exclude pre-eclampsia.
- Arrange an MSU to exclude a UTI.
- If the MSU is negative, exclude any underlying renal disease by checking serum creatinine and 24-hour urinary protein. (Proteinuria in pregnancy is defined as >300 mg/l.)
- Refer as appropriate.

ANAEMIA

The importance of severe anaemia during pregnancy is that perinatal mortality is increased and postpartum haemorrhage may become life-threatening.

Haemoglobin is measured routinely at booking, and at 28 and 34 weeks. The Hb concentration falls during pregnancy due to haemodilution. A low to normal Hb (10–11 g/dl) with a normal MCV and MCH suggests simple haemodilution. A pregnant woman is anaemic if the Hb is <10.

Management

Iron prophylaxis
This should be given to those at high risk of deficiency, e.g. those with: • a poor diet • closely spaced pregnancies • a past history of iron deficiency anaemia.

Folate prophylaxis
This should be given to all mothers at a dose of 400 µg per day up to 12 weeks of pregnancy. A higher dose of 5 mg per day should be given to mothers with a previous spina bifida child or a family history of spina bifida, as well as to mothers with: • a past history of folate deficiency • malabsorption • haemoglobinopathies • anticonvulsant therapy, e.g. phenytoin • multiple pregnancies • grand multiparity.

Mild anaemia can initially be assumed to be secondary to iron deficiency and treated with e.g. Pregaday, one tablet daily (100 mg elemental iron as ferrous fumarate and 350 µg of folate). Check the Hb 2 weeks later. It should rise at the rate of 0.5 g/dl per week. If the response is poor, or if the anaemia is more severe, double the dose of Pregaday. Check 2 weeks later, and refer if the haemoglobin is <9.

RHESUS-NEGATIVE MOTHERS

Fifteen per cent of women are rhesus negative. If the baby is rhesus positive and foetal red cells cross into the maternal circulation, maternal antibodies are produced. These cross back to the foetus, causing haemolysis.

Management
- Take blood at booking, and at 28 and 36 weeks to screen for rhesus antibodies.
- Anti-D may be administered routinely to rhesus-negative mothers at specific times in the pregnancy (e.g. primips at 28 weeks, 34–36 weeks and at delivery). Check the local protocol.

Give 500 IU of anti-D immunoglobulin to all rhesus-negative women after:

- spontaneous abortion (if >12 weeks)
- termination of pregnancy
- amniocentesis
- ectopic pregnancy
- antepartum haemorrhage
- delivery.

PRE-ECLAMPSIA

Pre-eclampsia is suggested, after >20 weeks, by a BP above 140/90 or a rise in diastolic pressure of more than 20 mmHg from booking. The presence of proteinuria is an additional indication of pre-eclampsia. Pretibial or generalised oedema may also be present.

Arrange urgent hospital assessment. If the mother is not admitted, the hospital will advise on frequency of follow-up.

ABNORMAL LIE

An oblique or transverse lie or breech presentation should be referred for hospital assessment from 34 weeks for discussion of possible trial of external cephalic version and/or mode of delivery.

HIGH HEAD

A 'high head' (i.e. one that lies totally outside the pelvis) is of less significance in a multiparous woman who has already experienced a vaginal delivery than in a primiparous woman. Before making this diagnosis, ensure that the bladder is empty. It is useful to ask the patient to lift her upper body onto her elbows. This may cause the head to descend. Refer primiparous women at 34 weeks for consultant assessment, and arrange an ultrasound to assess placental position. Multiparous women should be referred at 38 weeks for assessment of placental position, if not already known.

BACK PAIN

Back pain in pregnancy is usually lumbar, secondary to ligament laxity.

Management
- Advise on posture: try to eliminate, as far as possible, the lumbar lordosis when standing and sitting.
- Avoid heavy lifting.
- An elastic back support may be helpful (obtainable OTC or from the maternity physiotherapy department).
- Consider referral to maternity physiotherapy.

POSTPARTUM BLEEDING

The lochia usually disappear by 6 weeks. However, they may persist for some further weeks, but as long as they are decreasing and fading to pink or brown the patient can be reassured.

If the lochia remain red but bleeding is mild, consider using oral ergometrine 500 μg t.d.s. for 3 days. Co-amoxiclav 1 t.d.s. for 7 days may be useful in suspected endometritis (see below).

If bleeding is excessive (especially if there are clots present) or if the patient is pyrexial, admit with a view to ultrasound and/or ERPC.

POSTPARTUM PYREXIA

UTIs, DVTs and breast infections may present with pyrexia. Patients with endometritis (fever, foul discharge and low abdominal pain) should be admitted with a view to ERPC and/or intravenous antibiotics. (Foul lochia without fever can be treated at home with amoxycillin and metronidazole, or co-amoxiclav.)

POSTNATAL DEPRESSION

The maternity blues are considered to be normal. They are experienced by one-half to two-thirds of mothers, and usually occur in the first week. Postnatal depression, however, affects 10–15% of mothers, usually within the first 3 postnatal months.

Diagnosis
As with other forms of depression, the patient is not always aware that she is depressed, and diagnosis can be difficult. The Edinburgh Postnatal Depression Questionnaire is a useful screening tool which can be completed by all mothers. Women who score >9 should be assessed further.

Check for a physical cause, e.g. anaemia or hypothyroidism.

History

Risk factors for postnatal depression
- A past history of depression.
- A family history of depression.
- Problems in the early relationship between the patient and her own mother.
- Marital problems.
- Stressful life events.
- Emotional problems during the pregnancy.
- A first pregnancy.

Management
- The health visitor can play an important role in non-directive counselling. Encourage women to discuss their own needs separately from those of the baby.
- Antidepressants play an important role. Most are secreted in breast milk. Lofepramine 70–210 mg nocte is safe for breast-feeding mothers. The higher dose is often necessary.
- Consider involving other social support agencies, e.g. a social worker.
- Refer for counselling or to a psychiatrist, as appropriate.
- See depression (p. 294).

POSTNATAL CHECK

This takes place at 6 weeks. It is often the first time that the GP and the mother meet after the immediate postnatal period. It is a particularly important time to assess maternal mood.

Assessment

History Ask about:
- any continuing vaginal bleeding (persisting brown lochia is neither uncommon nor abnormal; see also p. 32)
- feelings about the birth and postnatal period
- sleep, mood, perineal discomfort, incontinence and breast- or bottle-feeding
- contraception
- rubella status.

Examination
- BP (especially if raised in pregnancy).
- Weight (if appropriate).
- Abdomen for muscle laxity. When divarication of the rectii muscles is significant (i.e. three or more fingers' breadths can be inserted between them), consider referral to a maternity physiotherapist.
- Breasts, especially if there are specific problems, e.g. sore nipples.
- Perineal wounds. Intercourse may already be pain-free, but there is often residual perineal soreness and tenderness.
- If a cervical smear is due, it is ideally delayed until about 3 months postpartum.

Management
- See sections on breast-feeding (below) and postnatal depression (p. 33), if appropriate.

• Discuss the importance of long-term abdominal and pelvic-floor exercises. Consider referral to a maternity physiotherapist if pelvic-floor weakness is significant.

BREAST-FEEDING

Many early breast feeding problems, e.g. mastitis, sore nipples and infant colic, are likely to be due to a failure to position the baby correctly on the breast. Therefore, always ensure a good feeding position. The midwife and health visitor are best placed to advise. Encourage unrestricted, demand feeding in order to stimulate lactation, and advise the mother to avoid giving the baby additional water or supplementary feeds, if possible.

SORE OR CRACKED NIPPLES

• Check positioning: the nipple should be in the roof of the baby's mouth, thus avoiding friction from the tongue.
• Encourage continued suckling as far as possible.
• Creams, ointments and local treatments are probably not effective.
• Apply breast milk to sore nipples and allow them to dry.

ENGORGEMENT

• Check positioning.
• Encourage continued suckling.
• A good supportive bra is helpful.
• It is often helpful to express engorged breasts gently before feeds. This may be more comfortable in a warm bath.
• Cold compresses between feeds may be soothing.

BLOCKED DUCTS (CAUSING TENDER LUMPS)

• Check positioning.
• Feed on the tender breast first.
• Gentle massage of a hard lump while feeding may be helpful. The milk should be smoothed towards the nipple.

MASTITIS

• A segment of the breast is usually red and tender and the patient is often pyrexial.

- 50% of cases may be non-infective, i.e. related to poor positioning, engorgement or localised obstructions (see above).
- If appropriate, treat with flucloxacillin 500 mg q.d.s. for 5 days (or erythromycin if the patient is allergic to penicillin). Antibiotic treatment will alter the taste of the milk and may cause the baby to develop mild diarrhoea.

SUPPRESSION OF LACTATION

- Lactation is naturally suppressed within 5 days of the cessation of breast-feeding.
- Advise simple analgesia and good breast support only.
- If lactation needs to be stopped more quickly, e.g. after stillbirth, prescribe bromocriptine 2.5 mg daily for 2–3 days, then 2.5 mg b.d. for 14 days.

GYNAECOLOGY

PREMENSTRUAL SYNDROME

Diagnosis

The diagnosis of PMS requires that the symptoms occur only in a particular phase of the ovarian cycle, nearly always at some time between ovulation and the onset of full menstrual flow.

> The distinction between PMS and psychological disorders that become worse in the premenstrual phase is often difficult. Examination is unnecessary.

Management

Advice

- Support and reassurance are vital, as there is undoubtedly a strong placebo effect.
- A menstrual diary, kept for at least 3 months, is useful.
- Exercise should be encouraged. (Increased endorphin release may improve symptoms.)
- A healthy, well-balanced diet should be encouraged in order to maintain steady blood glucose levels.

Prescribing

- NSAIDs are useful for pain symptoms and often improve mood and bloating.
- Pyridoxine (vitamin B_6) 10 mg per day from day 14 to the onset of menstruation is often used initially. Its efficacy is in doubt. It is prescribable on FP10 (GP10 in Scotland), and available OTC.
- Evening primrose oil (gamolenic acid) as a daily dose may be recommended. It is available OTC.
- Oestrogens may be used. (The rationale for their use is that cyclical ovarian activity is necessary for the symptoms of PMS, and oestrogens may suppress ovulation.)
  - The COC may be given. (Symptoms occasionally become worse.)
  - Transdermal oestradiol patches (25–100 μg) may be used twice a week, or consider an oestradiol implant (100 mg). Give concomitant treatment with a progestogen, e.g. norethisterone, 5 mg per day from day 19 to day 26, to prevent endometrial hyperplasia. Sequential combined oestrogen/progestogen patches are available.
- Progesterone and progestogens are often used, but there is no evidence of benefit. Treatment is given during the luteal phase only.
  - Natural progesterone has poor oral absorption and is therefore given PR or PV (100–800 mg daily), or transdermally as a cream.

- – Synthetic progestogens (oral), e.g. dydrogesterone 10 mg b.d. or norethisterone 5 mg t.d.s. may be given. (The POP may be helpful.)
- SSRIs often help to relieve all aspects of PMS.
- Diuretics can be helpful for fluid retention in the luteal phase.
- Bromocriptine 2.5 mg o.d. in the luteal phase can be helpful for cyclical breast pain.

INTERMENSTRUAL (OR POSTCOITAL) BLEEDING

Single episodes of non-menstrual bleeding are often innocent; the patient can usually be reassured and reviewed if the bleeding is persistent.

Persistent non-menstrual bleeding suggests a carcinoma until proven otherwise.

Diagnosis

History Ask about:
- The duration of symptoms.
- The amount and pattern of bleeding, e.g. postcoital, sporadic or regular.
- Contraception: if the woman is on the COC or the POP, query her compliance.
- The possibility of pregnancy.

Examination Examine the cervix and perform a smear and bimanual examination.

Investigations Arrange a pregnancy test, if appropriate.

Management
- Ask about STI risk factors (see p. 2) and consider *Chlamydia screening* (see p. 46) (Infection with *Chlamydia* may cause a blood-stained discharge.) Consider referral to a GUM clinic.
- If the woman is on the COC and she has experienced BTB for more than 3 months, consider changing her pill to one with a higher progestogen content.
- If there is an IUCD in situ consider removing it if the symptoms persist for more than 3 months.
- Spotting may occur for up to 6 months after IUS insertion.
- Cervical erosions, if symptomatic, e.g. causing postcoital bleeding, can be treated with a silver nitrate stick, prescribable on FP10 (GP10 in Scotland), or referred for treatment.

- Cervical polyps can be twisted and avulsed and sent for histology. Silver nitrate may be used on the resultant raw area. Always consider referral, especially if the base of the polyp is endocervical.

 Women over 40 should always be referred, unless the bleeding settles after removal of the presumed cause, e.g. a polyp. All women should be referred if the bleeding is persistent.

POSTMENOPAUSAL BLEEDING

Postmenopausal bleeding is any bleeding which occurs 1 year after the LMP.

Diagnosis

Examination Examine the vagina for, e.g. atrophic vaginitis, and the cervix, and perform a bimanual examination. Take a cervical smear, if appropriate.

Management
Women taking HRT should be referred for any significant unscheduled bleeding or consider review after stopping HRT.

Always refer to exclude malignancy, unless the bleeding is due to vaginitis which improves with treatment.

IRREGULAR PERIODS

Irregular periods are almost always a non-pathological variant of normal. They are most common at the extremes of reproductive life. The patient can usually be reassured. Irregular periods are a feature of POS (see p. 49). This symptom may progress to amenorrhoea (see p. 43).

DYSMENORRHOEA

Dysmenorrhoea, or painful menstruation, is common and can be severe, causing absence from school or work. It is usually fairly easy to differentiate between primary and secondary dysmenorrhoea.

PRIMARY DYSMENORRHOEA

(i.e. There is no pelvic pathology.)

Diagnosis

History
- It is common in young girls.
- It usually appears within 12 months of the menarche.
- Pain tends to occur within the first 2 days of the period.

Management
- Prostaglandin synthetase inhibitors, e.g. mefenamic acid 250–500 mg t.d.s. or naproxen 250–500 mg b.d. are usually helpful.
- The COC is especially useful, particularly when contraception is required.

SECONDARY DYSMENORRHOEA

(i.e. The dysmenorrhoea is associated with pelvic pathology, e.g. endometriosis, pelvic inflammatory disease or adenomyosis.)

Diagnosis

History
- The dysmenorrhoea usually starts several years after the menarche.
- There is often a clear change in the degree and timing of the pain.
- The pain often starts well before the period and may continue throughout the period.
- Discuss the significance of the dysmenorrhoea and the effect of the pain on the patient's lifestyle, e.g. time off work.

Examination Perform a speculum and bimanual examination to exclude any obvious pelvic pathology.

Management
- Consider removing an in situ IUCD.
- If the symptoms are suggestive of PID, perform an HVS and take endocervical swabs. (Include a chlamydial swab if available.) Treat with appropriate antibiotics and consider referral to a GUM clinic (see also p. 45).
- Patients should be referred in order to exclude pelvic pathology.

ENDOMETRIOSIS

Endometriosis is a common cause of dysmenorrhoea and pelvic pain. Diagnosis is by laparoscopy. Women with infertility and worsening symptoms should be referred. Hormonal treatment aims to suppress ovulation for

6–12 months, during which time the lesions atrophy. Endometriosis usually resolves at the menopause. Pelvic pain may be treated with:

- Prostaglandin synthetase inhibitors, e.g. mefenamic acid 250–500 mg t.d.s., p.r.n.
- The COC (usually one with a high progestogen content, e.g. Eugynon 30) may be prescribed with a pill-free break or continually.
- Progestogens, e.g. norethisterone 10–15 mg daily on a continuous basis.
- Danazol 200–800 mg daily, adjusted to achieve amenorrhoea. It inhibits gonadotrophin release. The dose can be titrated by balancing symptom control against side-effects, which are mainly androgenic.
- GnRH analogues, e.g. buserelin nasal spray 300 µg t.d.s. for a maximum of 6 months, produce a reversible artificial menopause.
- Surgery, e.g. local excision/diathermy of endometriotic tissue, or total hysterectomy and bilateral salpingo-oophorectomy may be considered.

MENORRHAGIA

Menorrhagia (regular heavy periods) is common at the extremes of reproductive life. Regular bleeding is relatively unlikely to be due to pelvic pathology.

Diagnosis

History Ask about: • the passing of clots • symptoms of anaemia.

Examination and investigations
- Check the haemoglobin.
- Perform a pelvic examination to exclude an organic cause, e.g. an ovarian or uterine tumour. Arrange a pelvic ultrasound scan if appropriate.
- Check the serum FSH if the menopause is suspected.

Management

Treatment
- Advise the woman to keep a menstrual diary.
- If there is an IUCD in situ, consider its removal.

Prescribing
- Antifibrinolytics, e.g. tranexamic acid 1–1.5 g t.d.s. or q.d.s. at the start of heavy bleeding for 3–4 days.
- Mefenamic acid 250–500 mg t.d.s: this should be taken during the worst few days of the period (it is used mainly for pain, and can be used in conjunction with tranexamic acid).
- COC: pills with a high progestogen content are more effective.

- To control torrential bleeding: prescribe norethisterone up to 10 mg t.d.s. The bleeding should stop within 48 hours. The dose can then be reduced to 5 mg b.d. for 12 days. The patient will experience a bleed on stopping treatment.
- The IUS should be considered, particularly for women also requiring contraception (see p. 16).

Referral If there is no response to treatment or if symptoms warrant it, consider referral for transcervical resection of the endometrium (TCRE), endometrial laser ablation (ELA) or hysterectomy.

Menorrhagia: referral criteria
Refer all women for gynaecological assessment if:

- They are aged >40 years (younger women are less likely to have an organic cause for their menorrhagia).
- The onset of menorrhagia is sudden.
- There is a suggestion of an organic cause (e.g. an ovarian or uterine tumour, endometriosis, pelvic inflammatory disease).

AMENORRHOEA

A woman with absent periods is usually concerned about abnormal body function and future fertility, or about possible pregnancy.

Primary amenorrhoea (i.e. when the menarche has not started by the age of 16 years):
- Congenital abnormalities usually present as primary amenorrhoea.
- Examine the external genitalia, and look for the development of secondary sexual characteristics.
- Check weight to exclude anorexia nervosa.
- Refer to a gynaecologist.

Secondary amenorrhoea The usual cause is recent rapid weight loss, emotional upset or post-hormonal contraception, i.e. hypothalamic. (A common scenario is a young student starting college, having left home.) Always exclude pregnancy. The cause is otherwise nearly always hormonal.

Diagnosis

History Ask about:
- date of the menarche
- LMP
- the normal cycle

- weight loss/eating disorder/stress
- drugs (e.g. the COC)
- galactorrhoea (this occurs in hyperprolactinaemia)
- menopausal symptoms (e.g. premature ovarian failure)
- hirsutism (this occurs in polycystic ovarian syndrome)
- general health (symptoms of, e.g. hypothyroidism, might be elicited).

Investigations
- Serum prolactin (raised in hyperprolactinaemia).
- Serum FSH/LH (raised in premature menopause).
- Serum testosterone (slightly raised, along with LH and sometimes prolactin, in polycystic ovarian syndrome).
- TFTs.

Management
- If blood tests are normal, amenorrhoea can be assumed to be hypothalamic and the woman can be reassured that her periods will return.
- Secondary amenorrhoea due to anorexia nervosa should be referred appropriately.
- Contraception should be discussed, if appropriate. If the patient is trying to become pregnant, consider referral and/or treatment with clomiphene (see p. 61).
- If blood tests are abnormal, refer as appropriate.

PELVIC PAIN

Diagnosis
Try to exclude the following diagnoses on history and examination:

- Appendicitis.
- Ectopic pregnancy: consider this in all sexually active women with pelvic pain. If appropriate, do an immediate pregnancy test and arrange an urgent pelvic ultrasound (a negative pregnancy test does not always exclude an ectopic pregnancy). Arrange immediate referral if in doubt.
- A ruptured ovarian cyst.
- Acute pelvic inflammatory disease.
- Other pelvic pathology, e.g. endometriosis. (This last should always be considered when recurrent episodes of pelvic pain fail to respond to antibiotic treatment.)

Management of acute pelvic inflammatory disease
Perform an HVS, and endocervical and urethral swabs. (Include a chlamydial swab if available.)

Treatment with antibiotics is usually given without a definite diagnosis, and should cover *Neisseria gonorrhoeae* and *Chlamydia* (the two major causes), and mixed aerobic and anaerobic infections. Treat with ofloxacin 400 mg b.d. and metronidazole 400 mg b.d. for 14 days. If gonococci are isolated, a single dose of ciprofloxacin 500 mg or ofloxacin 400 mg should be given.

Patients should be referred if the pain is severe, or the response to treatment is poor. IUCDs can be left in situ during treatment unless the infection is severe or persistent. Sexual contacts should be treated with doxycycline 100 mg o.d. for 10 days. Always seriously consider referral to a genitourinary clinic. Admit the patient if symptoms are severe.

VAGINAL DISCHARGE

The most common causes of vaginal discharge in general practice are *Candida* and *Gardnerella* (see also STIs, p. 46). All cases of vaginal discharge should be examined to exclude, e.g. a cervical erosion or foreign body, and an HVS should be taken. Endocervical and urethral swabs should be taken if sexual transmission is a possibility.

(All men with a urethral discharge should be referred to the local GUM clinic.)

CANDIDA

Candida is usually harboured by the woman, but can be sexually transmitted. The classic symptom is pruritis. The curdy white discharge may be minimal. It is often associated with dysuria and dyspareunia.

Management
Treat with an imidazole, e.g. clotrimazole pessaries (available OTC) 200 mg at night for 3 nights. Clotrimazole 1% cream can be used in addition for vulval pruritis.

Suggestions for recurrent symptoms, which are common:

- Give out patient information leaflets (e.g. with suggestions on avoiding nylon underwear and tights, and perfumed soaps).
- Treat the partner concurrently.
- Consider systemic oral antifungals, e.g. fluconazole in a single dose of 150 mg.
- Give intermittent prophylactic treatment, e.g. an imidazole pessary once a week.
- If *Candida* is caused by antibiotics, use prophylactic pessaries.
- If it is related to intercourse, insert a pessary after intercourse.
- Exclude diabetes, if appropriate.

If a recurrent discharge has previously been diagnosed by culture as either *Candida* or *Gardnerella*, treatment may reasonably be given 'blind', and swabs performed only if symptoms do not resolve.

GARDNERELLA (BACTERIAL VAGINOSIS)

Gardnerella is not considered to be sexually transmitted. The discharge is usually fishy-smelling, and may be seen as grey or yellow, watery and frothy.

Management
- Metronidazole 400 mg b.d. for 7 days.
- If symptoms are recurrent it may be worth treating the partner concurrently.

SEXUALLY TRANSMITTED INFECTIONS

In all STIs the partner should also be treated and sexual intercourse should be avoided until treatment is complete. Other recent sexual partners should be advised to seek medical advice.

Investigations should be performed to exclude the presence of any other STI. GUM clinics are best placed to arrange this, together with treatment of sexual contacts. See page 2 for considering possible STI risk.

TRICHOMONAS

The discharge is usually frothy and yellow.

Management
Metronidazole 400 mg b.d. for 7 days.

CHLAMYDIA

See also page 14.

Chlamydia is a major cause of PID, tubal infertility and ectopic pregnancy. It is the commonest curable STI in the industrialised world. Most women with *Chlamydia* are asymptomatic. Isolation requires cell culture methods which are not always available to GPs. Endocervical and urethral swabs should be taken using *Chlamydia* swabs. Standard regimens for treatment of PID will cover *Chlamydia* (see p. 45). Refer to a GUM clinic.

Management
- Doxycycline 100 mg b.d. for 7 days or erythromycin 500 mg b.d. for 14 days or azithromycin 1 g as a single dose.
- A test of cure investigation should be performed after treatment.

GONORRHOEA

Gonorrhoea is a major cause of PID. Patients should be referred to a GUM clinic.

Management
- Treatment should be coordinated by the GUM clinic.
- Treat with e.g. single-dose ciprofloxacin 500 mg or oflaxacin 400 mg.

GENITAL WARTS

Genital warts are diagnosed by clinical appearance. Patients should be referred to a GUM clinic for screening for other STIs.

Management
- Podophyllin paint applied only to the warts. (Podophyllin should be avoided in pregnancy.) Re-apply every 3–7 days.
- Consider cryotherapy as an alternative treatment for external warts.
- Annual smears are recommended after a diagnosis of genital warts.

GENITAL HERPES

Genital herpes is usually diagnosed by symptoms and clinical appearance. Patients should know that one-third of genital herpes infections are acquired from a mouth lesion rather than via sexual contact, that the delay between contact and symptoms may be long, e.g. years, and that they are more likely than not never to have a further attack. A swab of suspicious lesions should be sent in viral transport medium.

Advice Salt water baths and ice packs are helpful for painful lesions.

Management
- Analgesia, as appropriate.
- Treat with e.g. valaciclovir 500 mg b.d. for 5 days started as early as possible, but certainly within 7 days of the onset of symptoms.

Treatment of recurrent symptoms Depending on the degree of severity, the following may be used: simple analgesia alone, aciclovir cream or oral valaciclovir (as above) within 48 hours of onset, or, if recurrences are severe or frequent, continuous low-dose oral aciclovir 200–400 mg b.d. may be prescribed, usually on consultant advice.

> ⚠️ **A pregnant woman with a past history of genital herpes should have viral swabs taken in late pregnancy, as neonatal herpes can occur even when the mother has no overt signs of herpes.**

HIV AND AIDS

See page 192.

URETHRAL SYNDROME

In the urethral syndrome, symptoms of cystitis are present without a demonstrable UTI (i.e. an MSU shows $<10^5$ organisms per millilitre, or is sterile). Symptoms are usually mild and self-limiting, but may be recurrent. Patients are often anxious, and need reassurance.

Management

- The advice is similar to that for self-management of UTIs (see p. 65):
  - avoid scented soaps, bubble baths, etc.
  - alkalinise the urine with, e.g. sodium bicarbonate or potassium citrate mixture.
- It is worth considering treatment with an antibiotic, e.g. trimethoprim 200 mg b.d. for 3 days.
- Exclude intermittent infections by arranging MSUs, as appropriate.
- If the symptoms persist and are severe, refer to a urologist.

HIRSUTISM

In the vast majority of cases hirsutism is constitutional, especially in southern European women. Most hirsute women have increased androgen metabolism, at the high end of the spectrum of normality.

Diagnosis

Consider the following:

- a drug-related cause (e.g. phenytoin, corticosteroids, androgenic COC)
- a generalised endocrine disorder (e.g. hypothyroidism, Cushing's disease, acromegaly)

- inappropriate androgen production (raised serum testosterone and reduced SHBG) and polycystic ovarian syndrome (see below).

Management

Referral Consider referral to an endocrinologist or to a gynaecologist if:
- the above apply
- galactorrhoea is present
- the hirsutism is worsening rapidly.

Advice If investigations are normal and there are no associated features:
- Advise on cosmetic treatments (e.g. shaving, bleaching, waxing, depilatory creams, electrolysis). Electrolysis can be obtained on the NHS in severe cases.
- Encourage weight loss, if appropriate (serum testosterone levels increase with increasing weight).

Prescribing
- COC (particularly Dianette).
- Consider referral for treatment with high-dose cyproterone acetate.

POLYCYSTIC OVARIAN SYNDROME

The features of this common syndrome are polycystic ovaries on ultrasound together with irregular or absent periods and signs of excess androgens. Twenty per cent of asymptomatic women are found to have polycystic ovaries on ultrasound without the features of the syndrome. POS is thought to be related to insulin resistance. The patient often presents in her late teens or early twenties with some or all of the following symptoms: • obesity • virilisation with acne and hirsutes • irregular or absent periods • infertility (ovulation is sporadic or absent).

Investigations Blood results may show: raised LH, increased LH/FSH ratio, raised prolactin and raised testosterone. Ultrasound shows characteristic ovaries. Also check fasting blood sugar and serum cholesterol (POS patients have higher rates of IHD, hypertension and diabetes).

Management

Advice
- Lose weight.
- Encourage exercise, a healthy diet and advise against smoking.
- Discuss contraception, which is still necessary, if appropriate.
- Consider referral to a gynaecologist for assessment.

Prescribing
- Treat hirsutism, if appropriate (see p. 48).
- Treat acne, if appropriate (see p. 123).
- Regulate bleeding and prevent endometrial overstimulation with the COC (e.g. Dianette).
- Clomiphene will induce ovulation (see infertility, p. 60).
- Metformin improves insulin sensitivity, menstrual disturbance and ovulatory function. Seek specialist advice.

BREAST SCREENING

The government-funded National Breast Screening Programme offers routine 3-yearly mammography to all women aged 50–64, by invitation. Women aged 65 and over may receive 3-yearly mammography, but only on request.

The screening programme is reducing breast cancer mortality by 20–40%. No significant reduction in mortality has been shown in women under 50 years of age, following screening.

Mammography is not a tool for investigating established breast lumps.

BREAST AWARENESS

Most breast cancers are discovered by women themselves. Routine, formalised breast self-examination following a specific technique is no longer advocated, as it has not been shown to reduce breast cancer mortality and can cause considerable unnecessary anxiety. A more general breast awareness should be promoted. This encourages women to recognise what is normal, to know what changes to look out for, and to seek medical advice about these changes without delay.

In terms of teaching breast awareness, the practice nurse can do this opportunistically, but an ideal time is when women attend for either a well-woman check or a smear test. It is important to remember that men also need to be aware of changes in their breast tissue, as approximately 250 men in the UK develop breast cancer each year.

Advice
- Become familiar with the normal breast tissue and how it changes at different times of the month.
- Get into the habit of looking at and feeling the breasts from time to time.
- One way of looking at breasts is in a mirror, so that they can be seen from different angles.

- Feeling breasts is sometimes easier with a soapy hand in the bath or shower.
- Breasts go through many normal changes throughout life. They are affected by hormonal changes during the menstrual cycle, pregnancy, breast-feeding and the menopause, and by weight loss or weight gain.
- Breasts often become enlarged, tender and lumpy premenstrually. Some women may have tender lumpy breasts throughout their cycle.
- Breast tissue changes after the menopause and may become less dense, firm and more fatty, making the breasts feel softer. With age, breasts may get smaller. HRT may cause breast tenderness and make breasts feel firmer.

Changes to be aware of
- A change in size – one breast may become noticeably larger or lower.
- A nipple may become inverted or change its shape or position.
- A rash may occur on or around the nipple.
- Discharge from one or both nipples.
- Puckering or dimpling of the skin.
- Swelling under the armpit or around the collar bone.
- A lump or thickening in the breast that feels different from the rest of the breast tissue.
- Constant pain in one part of the breast, or in the armpit.

Breast awareness five point code
Advise the patient to:

- know what is normal for them
- look and feel
- know what changes to look for
- report any changes without delay
- attend for breast screening if aged 50 or over.

BREAST LUMPS

See page 265.

THE MENOPAUSE/CLIMACTERIC

The menopause is the process of inevitable ovarian failure leading to oestrogen deficiency. The average age of onset is 50.

Diagnosis

History The diagnosis is usually made on the history alone. Ask about:
• bleeding pattern • flushes and sweats • vaginal dryness and dyspareunia
• psychological symptoms, e.g. anxiety and depression.

Investigations
• Consider a pregnancy test.
• Consider thyroid function tests.

Check serum FSH if the diagnosis is in doubt, e.g. in:

• hysterectomised women
• those already taking the COC or HRT (see p. 18) and experiencing regular withdrawal bleeds
• those experiencing amenorrhoea secondary to the POP
• those with oligomenorrhoea or amenorrhoea and menopausal symptoms under the age of 45.

Two serum FSH levels of >30 U/l 3 months apart are diagnostic of the menopause, but even a mildly raised level may be suggestive.

Management

Discuss: • the patient's understanding of the menopause • life changes and stresses • the prevention of cardiovascular disease and osteoporosis (see p. 249) • HRT (see below).

Hysterectomy with ovarian conservation is associated with early ovarian failure.

Bleeding usually becomes increasingly infrequent as the menopause approaches. However, any bleeding which occurs 1 year or more after the last period is considered to be postmenopausal (see p. 40) and should be referred for investigation to exclude malignancy.

⚠️ **Irregular, very heavy or painful bleeding should not be considered to be part of the normal menopause, and should be referred for endometrial biopsy.**

HORMONE REPLACEMENT THERAPY (HRT)

HRT is prescribed for menopausal symptoms (e.g. hot flushes, vaginal dryness and low mood) and for the prophylaxis of postmenopausal osteoporosis. It is recommended for perimenopausal and postmenopausal women who are symptomatic (ideal duration of use is at least 1 year) or are at high risk of osteoporosis (ideal duration of use is at least 5–10 years), especially for those who have had an early menopause.

Unopposed oestrogens overstimulate the endometrium. This can lead to endometrial hyperplasia and carcinoma of the endometrium. Only hysterectomised women may be treated with unopposed oestrogen. Women with an intact uterus should be treated with oestrogen/progestogen combinations.

Contraindications
- Oestrogen-sensitive malignancies (breast or endometrium).
- Major thromboembolic disease (in view of minor adverse effects on clotting factors and platelet function).
- Severe kidney or liver disease.
- Gall bladder disease.
- Otosclerosis (may worsen on HRT).

Advantages
- Treats overt symptoms.
- Prevents osteoporosis.

Disadvantages
- Regular bleeding in women with a uterus taking cyclical preparations. (The withdrawal bleed, lasts for several days, but is usually lighter than a normal period.)
- A small increased risk of breast carcinoma related to duration of use. Any excess risk disappears within about 5 years of stopping. About 32 in every 1000 women aged 50–65 years and not using HRT will have breast cancer diagnosed over 15–20 years. In those using combined HRT for 5 years this number rises by 6 extra cases in 1000 and by 19 extra cases in 1000 after 10 years use. In those using oestrogen-only HRT for 5 years breast cancer is diagnosed in about 1.5 extra cases in 1000, and 5 extra cases in 1000 after 10 years use. Tibolone increases the risk of breast cancer, but to a lesser extent than with combined HRT.
- Long-term treatment with HRT slightly increases the incidence of stroke, DVT and pulmonary embolism.

First appointment
History Ask about: • the date of the last period • hot flushes and sweats • depression, anxiety and mood changes • genitourinary problems, e.g. vaginal dryness, dyspareunia and urinary incontinence • risk factors for osteoporosis (see p. 249).

Hormone replacement therapy

Brand	Oestrogen	Progestogen	Formulation*	Bleed†	RX‡	Cost/28 days (£)
SYSTEMIC						
Sequential combined therapy						
Climagest	Oestradiol (1 mg, 2 mg)	Norethisterone (1 mg)	T	M	2	4.78
Cyclo-progynova	Oestradiol (1 mg, 2 mg)	Levo/norgestrel (0.25 mg/0.5 mg)	T	M	2	3.34
Elleste Duet	Oestradiol (1 mg, 2 mg)	Norethisterone (1 mg)	T	M	2	3.24
Estracombi	Oestradiol (50 μg)	Norethisterone (0.25 mg)	P	M	2	11.14
Evorel-Pak	Oestradiol (50 μg)	Norethisterone (1 mg)	P + T	M	2	8.45
Evorel Sequi	Oestradiol (50 μg)	Norethisterone (170 μg)	P	M	2	11.00
Femapak	Oestradiol (40 μg, 80 μg)	Dydrogesterone (10 mg)	P + T	M	2	8.45, 8.95
Femoston	Oestradiol (1 mg, 2 mg)	Dydrogesterone (10 mg)	T	M	2	4.99
Femoston 2/20	Oestradiol (2 mg)	Dydrogesterone (20 mg)	T	M	2	7.48
FemSeven Sequi	Oestradiol (50 μg)	Levonorgestrel (10 μg)	P	M	2	9.98
FemTab Sequi	Oestradiol (2 mg)	Levonorgestrel (75 μg)	T	M	2	5.05
Novofem	Oestradiol (1 mg)	Norethisterone (1 mg)	T	M	2	4.50
Nuvelle	Oestradiol (2 mg)	Levonorgestrel (75 μg)	T	M	2	5.05
Premique Cycle	Conj. oestrogens (0.625 mg)	Medroxyprogesterone (10 mg)	T	M	2	8.29
Prempak-C	Conj. oestrogens (0.625 mg, 1.25 mg)	Norgestrel (150 μg)	T	M	2	5.89
Tridestra	Oestradiol (2 mg)	Medroxyprogesterone (20 mg)	T	Q	2	7.93
Trisequens	Oestradiol (2 mg, 2 mg, 1 mg; 4 mg, 4 mg, 1 mg)	Norethisterone (1 mg)	T	M	2	4.80
Continuous combined therapy						
Climesse	Oestradiol (2 mg)	Norethisterone (0.7 mg)	T	X	—	8.62
Elleste Duet Conti	Oestradiol (2 mg)	Norethisterone (1 mg)	T	X	—	5.99
Evorel Conti	Oestradiol (50 μg)	Norethisterone (170 μg)	P	X	—	12.90
Femoston Conti	Oestradiol (1 mg)	Dydrogesterone (5 mg)	T	X	—	7.54
FemSeven Conti	Oestradiol (50 μg)	Levonorgestrel (7 μg)	P	X	—	12.90

FemTab Continuous	Oestradiol (2 mg)	Norethisterone (1 mg)	T	—	X	6.01
Indivina	Oestradiol (1 mg, 2 mg)	Medroxyprogesterone (2.5 mg, 5 mg)	T	—	X	7.54
Kliofem	Oestradiol (2 mg)	Norethisterone (1 mg)	T	—	X	5.15
Kliovance	Oestradiol (1 mg)	Norethisterone (0.5 mg)	T	—	X	5.15
Nuvelle Continuous	Oestradiol (2 mg)	Norethisterone (1 mg)	T	—	X	6.01
Premique	Conj. oestrogens (0.625 mg)	Medroxyprogesterone (5 mg)	T	—	X	9.05
Gonadomimetic						
Livial	Tibolone (2.5 mg)		T	—	X	13.05
Unopposed oestrogen (if uterus is intact an adjunctive progestogen must be used)						
Aerodiol	Oestradiol (150 µg)		S	—		7.25
Climaval	Oestradiol (1 mg, 2 mg)		T	—		2.55
Elleste Solo MX	Oestradiol (40 µg, 80 µg)		P	—		5.19, 5.99
Estraderm MX	Oestradiol (25 µg, 50 µg, 75 µg, 100 µg)		P	—		5.20, 5.22, 6.08, 6.31
Estraderm TTS	Oestradiol (25 µg, 50 µg, 100 µg)		P	—		6.21, 6.23, 7.52
Evorel	Oestradiol (25 µg, 50 µg, 75 µg, 100 µg)		P	—		3.07, 3.48, 3.70, 3.84
Fematrix	Oestradiol (40 µg, 80 µg)		P	—		5.50, 6.00
FemSeven	Oestradiol (50 µg, 75 µg, 100 µg)		P	—		4.57, 5.29, 5.52
FemTab	Oestradiol (1 mg, 2 mg)		T	—		2.57
Harmogen	Oestrone (0.93 mg)		T	—		3.00
Harmonin	Oestriol/oestradiol/oestrone (1 strength)		T	—		2.36
Menorest	Oestradiol (50 µg, 75 µg)		P	—		7.69, 8.95
Menoring	Oestradiol (50 µg)		VR	—		9.83
Oestrogel	Oestradiol (1.5 mg)		G	—		7.95

Continued

Hormone replacement therapy (contd)						
Brand	Oestrogen	Progestogen	Formulation*	Bleed†	RX‡	Cost/ 28 days (£)
Premarin	Conj. oestrogens (0.625 mg, 1.25 mg)		T		–	3.24, 4.40
Prognova	Oestradiol (1 mg, 2 mg)		T		–	2.57
Prognova TS	Oestradiol (50 μg, 100 μg)		P		–	5.96, 6.56
Sandrena	Oestradiol (0.5 mg, 1 mg)		G		–	5.68, 6.54
Zumenon	Oestradiol (1 mg, 2 mg)		T		–	2.55
Adjunctive progestogen						
Crinone		Progesterone (4%)	VG		–	11.08
Duphaston HRT		Dydrogesterone (10 mg)	T		–	1.05
Micronor HRT		Norethisterone (1 mg)	T		–	1.25
LOCAL						
Oestrogen only						
Estring	Oestradiol (7.5 μg)		VR		–	
Ortho-Gynest Pessary	Oestriol (0.5 mg)		P		–	
Ortho-Gynest Cream	Oestriol (0.01%)		VC		–	
Ovestin	Oestriol (0.1%)		VC		–	
Premarin	Conj. oestrogens (0.0625%)		VC		–	
Tampovagan	Stilboestrol (0.5 mg)		P		–	
Vagifem	Oestradiol (25 μg)		VT		–	

Reproduced from *Monthly Index for Medical Specialities* with permission from Haymarket Medical Ltd
* G, gel; P, patch; S, spray; T, tablet; VC, vaginal cream; VG, vaginal gel; VR, vaginal ring; VT, vaginal tablet
† M, monthly; Q, quarterly; X, no bleed
‡ Combination packs incur multiple prescription charges

Examination
- BP.
- Weight.
- Discuss breast awareness.
- Consider vaginal examination.
- Check smear status (3-yearly).
- Mammography should be arranged for women with a family history of breast cancer.

Advice
- Offer general advice relating to the menopause (see p. 51) and osteoporosis (see p. 249).
- Discuss contraception if appropriate (see p. 18). HRT is not a form of contraception.

Prescribing (The lowest effective maintenance dose should be prescribed.)
- Continuous daily oestrogen should be prescribed for hysterectomised women, e.g. Premarin 0.625–1.25 mg daily.
- Oestrogen/progestogen preparations should be prescribed for women with an intact uterus. Continuous oestrogen with 12–13 days of progestogen at the end of each monthly cycle, producing a regular monthly bleed, is commonly prescribed in the perimenopause, e.g. Nuvelle or Prempak-C. Amenorrhoeic regimens (using continuous combined oestrogen and progestogen) may be used for women who are at least 1 year postmenopausal, e.g. Premique or Kliofem. Irregular bleeding is a common side-effect of these regimens during the early treatment stages. If it continues, endometrial abnormality should be excluded, and consideration given to cyclical HRT instead.
- Oestrogen can be given as a subdermal implant, and renewed every few months as symptoms recur.
- Oestrogen can be given transdermally as a patch. (This avoids the first-pass effect through the liver and has a beneficial effect on lipids.) Patches are expensive compared to oral oestrogens.
- The low-dose COC alleviates perimenopausal symptoms. In fit non-smokers it can be prescribed up to the menopause.
- Tibolone combines weak oestrogenic, progestogenic and androgenic activity. It is useful for women who cannot take oestrogen, for osteoporosis prophylaxis and symptom control. It does not produce withdrawal bleeds, but spotting is a common side-effect.
- Vaginal oestrogen creams, e.g. ovestin, are useful for women with genitourinary problems who do not wish to take systemic HRT, or in whom HRT is contraindicated. They are, to some degree, systemically absorbed, and if they are used on a long-term basis some require oral progestogen for 10–14 days of each month to combat endometrial hyperplasia. Modified-release vaginal tablets and an impregnated vaginal ring are also available.

Follow-up

Follow-up should be at 3 months and subsequently 6-monthly or annually.

History

- Ask about any abnormal bleeding. (The bleeding pattern is commonly abnormal in the first 2–3 months, but should be regular subsequently.)
- Some women with an intact uterus do not experience a progestogen withdrawal bleed. This is not a cause for concern. Exclude pregnancy.

Examination

- B.P.
- Weight.
- Vaginal examination. (This is only necessary routinely in the presence of unscheduled bleeding.)
- Check the smear status.
- Check the mammogram status (see also p. 50).

CERVICAL CYTOLOGY

Cervical screening is the process of taking a sample of cells from the cervix to look for possible precancerous changes in asymptomatic women. It is an example of secondary prevention. Practice nurses carry out the majority of cervical screeing in general practice, but other community nurses may do so in family planning or cytology clinics. Other primary care nurses may be involved in giving information about the programme in order to encourage attendance.

The most important aspect of successful cervical screening is ensuring that the correct cells are collected in the sample, and it is therefore important that all nurses carrying out this procedure receive appropriate training as part of the National Health Service Cervical Screening Programme (NHSCSP).

Taking a smear is an invasive procedure for which consent should always be obtained.

It is important when inviting women for a smear test that they are advised not to have a bath or shower immediately prior to attendance and to refrain from intercourse in the preceeding 24 hours.

If it is difficult to view the cervix because of its posterior position, asking the women to place her two fists under her buttocks to tilt her pelvis upwards usually facilitates a good view, which is essential in order to take an adequate smear. In obese women, asking the woman to lay in a left lateral position and using a Simms speculum should overcome any difficulty.

Liquid based cytology is a new method of collecting and preparing cell samples from a woman's cervix. Samples are collected using a brush-like device rather than a spatula. The head of the brush is rinsed or broken off into a container of preservative fluid that protects the cervical cells. The container is then sent to the laboratory for examination. The evidence shows that this method may result in better quality samples that are easier to read, and thus reduce the number of tests that need to be repeated.

Discussion points for primary prevention of cervical cancer

- Stopping or reducing smoking lessens the risk of cervical cancer.
- An increased number of sexual partners (for both men and women) increases the risk.
- Patients should avoid intercourse with partners with genital warts, unless a condom is used.
- Barrier methods of contraception are probably protective.

National screening guidelines

- All women aged 20–64, who have at any time been sexually active, should be screened at least every 5 years.
- Screening is unnecessary for women who have never been sexually active.
- Women aged 65 or over who have had regular negative smears do not need further screening. Women aged 65 or over who have never had a smear should be encouraged to have one.
- Instructions for follow-up or colposcopy referral will be given on smear reports.

Negative smear reports sometimes reveal incidental findings which require action as follows:

Specific infections
- *Trichomonas*: treat (see p. 46).
- *Candida*: treat if symptomatic (see p. 45).
- *Actinomyces*-like organisms (ALOs): these may colonise the genital tract in the presence of an IUCD. If the woman is asymptomatic, discuss the possible risk of pelvic infection. Leave the IUCD in situ and arrange 6-monthly follow-ups, including bimanual examination. Alternatively, remove or exchange the device (this usually leads to disappearance of ALOs) and repeat the smear after 6 months. If the woman is symptomatic (i.e. pelvic pain, dyspareunia or discharge), remove the IUCD, send the threadless device for culture and take an endocervical swab. If ALOs are

found, treat with high-dose penicillin (2–3 g per day) or erythromycin for at least 2 weeks. Arrange an alternative method of contraception.
- Herpes simplex: no action.
- Inflammatory changes: no action, or consider taking an HVS and chlamydial swabs and treat as appropriate.

Indications for performing a non-routine cervical smear
- Intermenstrual bleeding.
- Postcoital bleeding.
- A suspicious-looking cervix.

> Clinical suspicion of cervical pathology should prompt referral for colposcopy, even if a cervical smear is normal.

INFERTILITY

> Infertility is common, affecting about 15% of couples. It is important to note that 25% of cases of infertility remain unexplained.

The main causes of infertility are: • disorders of spermatogenesis • ovulation disorders • tubal/pelvic pathology • others, e.g. endometriosis, sperm/mucus problems.

Diagnosis

History
- Confirm regular intercourse during the fertile period. The fertile period is from day 8 to day 17 in a normal 28-day cycle (see calendar method, p. 16).
- Ninety per cent of women of proven fertility will conceive within 12 months. Investigation is therefore not usually undertaken until the couple have been attempting to conceive for 12 months or more. The couple should ideally be seen together.

Investigations Before referral, the GP can arrange for semen analysis (see p. 61) and confirm ovulation.

Confirmation of ovulation Ovulation is suggested by: • regular periods • premenstrual symptoms • ovulation pain.
Ovulation can be confirmed by:

- Basal body temperature: this rises by 0.2–0.5°C after ovulation. Basal temperature thermometers can be prescribed on an FP10 (GP10 in

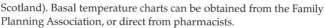
Scotland). Basal temperature charts can be obtained from the Family Planning Association, or direct from pharmacists.

- Mid-luteal phase serum progesterone of >30 nmol/l. The blood test should be taken about 8 days before the next period is due (usually day 19 to day 21).
- Urinary LH kits: these can be bought OTC. They detect the LH surge in mid-cycle.

Semen analysis
A fresh warm specimen, produced after 48 hours of abstinence, should be examined in the laboratory within 2 hours of production.
Normal values:

- volume >2 ml
- count >20 million/ml
- motility >50%
- normal morphology >50%.

Management
Clomiphene may be given to women who have been shown not to be ovulating, while awaiting hospital assessment. Their partner must have a normal semen analysis. Prescribe clomiphene 50 mg daily for 5 days starting on day 2. Ovulation can be confirmed by a rise in day 19 to day 21 progesterone. In the absence of ovulation, a second course of 100 mg daily for 5 days can be given. Three courses constitute an adequate therapeutic trial.

TERMINATION OF PREGNANCY REQUEST

Most TOPs are performed under point 2 (see box overleaf).

Assessment

History Ask about:
- Circumstances of pregnancy and request for TOP.
- Last menstrual period and calculate gestation. (Was the LMP normal?)
- Usual cycle.
- Date of last smear.
- Past history of STI.
- Previous births, miscarriages or pregnancy terminations.

Investigations Carry out a pregnancy test. (Confirmation of the pregnancy should not usually be a cause for delay in referral.)

The 1967 Abortion Act (revised in 1991) allows the following grounds for termination of pregnancy:

1. risk to the life of the woman or risk of grave permanent physical or mental injury to the woman (no time limit)
2. risk of injury to the physical or mental health of the woman (only legal up to 24 weeks)
3. risk of injury to the physical or mental health of existing child(ren) (only legal up to 24 weeks)
4. substantial risk of the child being born with serious abnormalities (no time limit).

Management
- Help the woman to make a decision about the future of her pregnancy.
- Give information about the different methods of TOP, if appropriate, and refer to a gynaecologist:
  - surgical treatment
  - medical treatment with RU486 (mifepristone) and prostaglandins (only suitable for use in pregnancies of less than 9 weeks' gestation).
- Discuss future contraceptive plans.
- Arrange follow-up 2 weeks after the termination.

Administration
Fill in form HSA1 and send with referral letter.

CHAPTER 4

UROGENITAL MEDICINE

URINARY TRACT INFECTION (UTI)

The average GP with a list of 2000 patients will see 30–40 cases of UTI a year. UTIs are particularly common in sexually active women, older menopausal women and men with prostatic hypertrophy. They usually present with urinary frequency, dysuria and cloudy urine, and sometimes suprapubic or loin pain or tenderness, haematuria, fever and even rigors. Up to half of all non-pregnant women with symptoms of lower UTI have no detectable bacterial infection, and therefore drug treatment is often unnecessary.

Diagnosis

History Ask about: • the above symptoms • previous history of UTI • form of contraception.

Some other causes of UTI symptoms
- Atrophic vaginitis.
- Trauma from intercourse.
- Bladder outlet obstruction, e.g. prostatism.
- Soreness from e.g. deodorants.
- Bacteria which are difficult to culture, e.g. *Chlamydia* and *Gardnerella*.
- Urethral syndrome (see p. 48).

Examination Examination is usually unnecessary, but look for suprapubic or loin tenderness, if appropriate.

Investigations
- Dipstick urine to test for protein, nitrite (a bacterial metabolite) and leucocytes.
- Send an MSU for microscopy, culture and antibiotic sensitivities (this is not always essential before starting treatment). The MSU must show a pure growth in excess of 10^5 organisms/ml and white cells in excess of $50/mm^3$ in order to confirm a significant infection.

The following groups should always have an MSU sent for culture:

1. pregnant women
2. children
3. men
4. catheterised patients
5. patients who have failed to respond to initial antibiotic treatment
6. patients with persistent symptoms.

Management

Advise the patient to drink copious fluids, especially alkaline liquids, e.g. sodium bicarbonate or potassium citrate mixture.

Proteinuria and haematuria have many causes other than UTI. Negative urine tests for leucocytes and nitrite can reliably indicate that a UTI is not present.

First-line treatment of UTIs

Females with simple UTI Trimethoprim 200 mg b.d. or amoxycillin 250 mg t.d.s. for 3 days.

Children aged >12, men, and women with clinical evidence of renal involvement (e.g. fever, loin pain) Trimethoprim 200 mg b.d. or amoxycillin 250 mg for 7–10 days. (Check dosage for young children.)

UTI in pregnancy Cephalexin 1 g b.d. for 7–10 days, or nitrofurantoin MR 100 mg b.d. for 7–10 days.

Management of recurrent UTIs in women

- If recurrent symptoms are due to the same organism, ensure that treatment is with an antibiotic to which the pathogen has been shown to be sensitive, check compliance and continue the antibiotic for 5 7 days.
- Discuss, if appropriate:
  – using a lubricant with intercourse
  – passing urine after intercourse
  – improving perineal hygiene
  – avoiding tight clothing
  – avoiding scented soaps, bubble bath, etc.
  – drinking lots of fluid
  – contraception (e.g. a diaphragm may encourage UTIs).
- Consider arranging a plain abdominal X-ray (to look for radio-opaque stones), followed by an ultrasound scan of the urinary tract or an IVU to exclude renal cortical scars from previous infections, or evidence of obstruction.
- If these investigations are normal, consider giving prophylactic antibiotics. One-quarter of the usual 24-hour dose should be given at night and continued until the urine has been sterile for 1 year, e.g. trimethoprim 100 mg nocte. Before starting on this regimen, consider referral for urological assessment.
- Patients whose UTIs are clearly related to intercourse may take a single dose of antibiotic within 2 hours of intercourse.
- Exclude diabetes.
- Consider prescribing a 'spare' course of antibiotics for the patient to start at the onset of symptoms.

UTIs in men See management of UTIs in general (p. 65). Refer men with a confirmed UTI to a urologist.

Men with symptoms of a UTI but no infection may have prostatitis. They usually have discomfort behind the testicles. Prostatitis can be diagnosed by sending the first urine of the morning (the early part of the stream) for microscopy and confirming the presence of threads of white cells. Treat with ciprofloxacin 500 mg b.d. or trimethoprim 200 mg b.d. for 28 days, or longer if the symptoms have not completely settled.

UTIs in children See page 86.

PROTEINURIA

A trace of proteinuria on dipstick, in the absence of microscopic haematuria, is nearly always benign.

Management
- Exclude fever or recent exercise.
- Dipstick urine for nitrite, leucocytes and blood.
- Arrange MSU.
- Check BP.
- Arrange 24 hour urine collection for total protein excretion (150 mg is the upper limit of normal), if appropriate.
- Arrange bloods for U&E, creatinine and fasting blood sugar, if appropriate.

> A patient with persistent proteinuria (i.e. dipstick positive for protein recorded on three separate urine samples, including an early morning urine) with or without microscopic haematuria, should be referred to a urologist for consideration of renal imaging/biopsy.

URINARY STONES

Ureteric colic usually presents with very severe unilateral loin pain, often accompanied by vomiting. The diagnosis is confirmed by the presence of microscopic haematuria. Patients with undiagnosed backache or vague loin pain may be harbouring a stone.

Diagnosis
Investigations (These are only necessary with the first stone.)

Urgent
- Urinalysis (for blood).
- Arrange an urgent IVU during an episode of pain. This will indicate the exact location of any stone, the function of both kidneys and the presence of any obstruction.

Less urgent
- MSU for microscopy and culture.
- A plain abdominal X-ray (90% of urinary stones are radio-opaque) and ultrasound scan.
- Bloods should be arranged by the GP or the hospital, depending on the situation:
  - FBC and ESR
  - U&E, creatinine and urate
  - calcium, phosphate and alkaline phosphatase.
- Chemical analysis of the stone, if appropriate.

Management

Treatment
- Some patients improve immediately without intervention due to spontaneous passing of the stone.
- Give diclofenac 75 mg i.m. (or 100 mg PR) or pethidine 100 mg i.m., together with prochlorperazine 12.5 mg i.m., if required, for vomiting.
- Less severe pain can be controlled with e.g. oral NSAIDs or oral pethidine.
- Push fluids.

Referral Consider referring all patients with first-time stones for urgent urological assessment. Patients with the following should always be admitted:

- possible stones where the GP does not have access to imaging procedures
- obstruction on IVU
- large calculi which cannot be passed spontaneously
- ureteric colic that does not resolve quickly
- reduced renal function
- infection.

Patients with first-time stones who do not need urgent admission should be referred to the urology outpatient clinic.

URINARY INCONTINENCE

Incontinence is involuntary leakage of urine and is a common and disabling condition. It is estimated that as many as 60% of the elderly population and

40% of women over the age of 20 suffer from some form of urinary incontinence. It can be significantly improved by appropriate intervention, but is underdiagnosed because a large percentage of sufferers do not consult their doctor. Stress incontinence and urge incontinence (detrusor instability) are responsible for over 90% of cases of incontinence. The two often coexist, but the most useful distinguishing factor is the absence of urgency in stress incontinence.

Diagnosis

History It is important to take advantage of routine screening opportunities to identify sufferers, e.g. well-woman clinics, chronic disease follow-ups, postnatal clinics, etc.
  Ask about:

- Stress incontinence: leakage of urine with exercise, coughing or sneezing.
- Urge incontinence:
  - urinary frequency, day and night
  - hurrying to get to the toilet
  - not being able to get to the toilet in time.
- Overflow incontinence (bladder outflow obstruction):
  - difficulty passing urine (hesitancy)
  - dribbling after passing urine
  - poor stream
  - nocturia
  - a sensation of incomplete bladder-emptying.
- Passive incontinence:
  - passing urine without knowing it
  - accidents in bed at night.

General questions Ask about:
- Pain on passing urine (suggestive of UTI, atrophic vaginitis or obstruction).
- Liquid intake. Alcohol and coffee are diuretics.
- Drugs, e.g. diuretics, antidepressants.
- The use of pads or towels.
- Past history, e.g. stroke, dementia, Parkinson's disease, multiple sclerosis, prolapsed disc, spinal injury, previous pelvic surgery, obstetric history, etc.

Examination Look for: • constipation • a palpable bladder (overflow incontinence) • pelvic masses, e.g. fibroids • other local 'lumps', e.g. a large inguinal hernia • cystocoele • local infections, e.g. *Candida* • atrophic vaginitis • enlarged prostate • tight foreskin.
  Assess the pelvic floor muscles by asking the patient to pull up the pelvic floor while you are performing a pelvic examination.

Investigations
- Dipstick urine for blood, sugar, protein, nitrite and leucocytes.

- MSU, where appropriate, for microscopy, culture and antibiotic sensitivities.
- A urinary diary, documenting frequency and volume of urine passed, and drinks taken, can be helpful.

Management

Most patients can be treated satisfactorily by the GP.

Stress incontinence (due to weakness of the urethral sphincter)
- Encourage reduction of intra-abdominal pressure by:
  - reducing weight, if appropriate
  - stopping smoking, if appropriate
  - avoiding constipation
  - avoiding heavy lifting.
- Regular pelvic floor exercises (i.e. repetitive squeezing of the pelvic floor) improve tone and support. Tighten the front (bladder) and back (bowel) passages. Count to four slowly, then release slowly. Do this several times and repeat every hour or so, if possible. These exercises, which can be done at any time, and are not evident to others, should ideally be continued for life.
- Consider referral to a physiotherapist for instruction on pelvic floor exercises, treatment with graduated vaginal cones or electrical stimulation of the pelvic floor (faradism or interferential treatment).
- Consider referral for urodynamic investigations and/or surgery, e.g. colposuspension or tension-free vaginal tape (TVT) urethral sling, if:
  - the exact diagnosis is in doubt
  - conservative methods have failed
  - symptoms recur following surgery.
- Treat atrophic vaginitis with local oestrogen cream or systemic HRT.

Urge incontinence (due to detrusor instability)
- Bladder retraining involves encouraging the patient to void increasingly larger volumes of urine at less frequent intervals, thus relearning inhibition of abnormal detrusor muscle contractions.
- Drugs to stabilise the detrusor muscle can be used in addition to bladder retraining, e.g. oxybutynin 2.5–5 mg t.d.s. or tolteridone 1–2 mg b.d. (sustained release preparations reduce the anticholinergic side-effects). Once continence has been regained, many patients are able to sustain the improvement without medication.
- The patient may need psychological support.

Living with incontinence
- Refer to a district nurse for advice on appliances, e.g. incontinence pads.
- Consider involving local continence advisors.

PROSTATISM

Prostatism, or symptoms of outflow obstruction in men, is common, particularly in the elderly, and often not volunteered by the patient.

Diagnosis

History Ask about: • poor urinary stream • hesitancy • frequency • nocturia • terminal dribble • bone pain, which raises the possibility of malignant bony secondaries.

Examination Look for:
- The enlarged bladder of urinary retention, which can be painless in chronic retention.
- Enlargement of the prostate gland, by performing a digital rectal examination. (The detection of malignancy in the prostate by digital examination is possible only with experience of feeling normal prostates. As a general rule, the malignant prostate is hard, craggy, irregular and often enlarged, with the central sulcus obliterated.)

Investigations

All cases
- MSU, to exclude a UTI as cause of frequency.
- Blood for C&E, to exclude obstructive uropathy.
- Serum prostate specific antigen (PSA). A level greater than 4.0 raises the possibility of malignancy, but there are many false-positive results.

In suspected malignancy
- PSA will often be raised if there is clinical suspicion of malignancy.
- X-ray of a painful, bony area, e.g. the pelvis or hips, is a sensitive way of detecting bony secondaries.

Management
- Frequency and nocturia in benign prostatic hyperplasia may be helped by a selective alpha blocker, e.g. indoramin 20 mg b.d. (relaxes smooth muscle, producing an increase in urinary flow rate).
- Refer for urological opinion in suspected malignancy, obstructive uropathy or prostatism symptoms resistant to treatment.
- For the patient too infirm for surgery, incontinence aids may become necessary. Consider monitoring C&E in such patients, to detect obstructive uropathy.
- Catheterisation becomes necessary in acute retention, deteriorating renal function and as an alternative in incontinence control.

Patients significantly troubled by symptoms of prostatism should be offered referral, as a routine case, for consideration for surgery. Cases of malignancy, suspected on clinical or biochemical grounds, should be offered an urgent referral for tissue diagnosis.

Prevention/screening

There is much debate at present about the merits of screening for prostatic cancer. The three methods available are: • digital rectal examination • transrectal ultrasound scanning • serum PSA.

Although all methods should, in theory, enable the earlier detection of prostate problems, none has been shown so far to reduce mortality from prostate cancer.

TESTICULAR SELF-EXAMINATION (TSE)

Testicular cancer is the most common form of cancer in young men in the UK and occurs mostly in those aged 19–44 years. It is easily treated, particularly if detected at an early stage. Therefore it is important for healthcare professionals to use every opportunity to explain to men the importance of regular self-checking to help in early detection of the disease.

Advice
- From the time of puberty onwards, do a simple regular check to help recognise what is normal; this will enable the detection of any changes at an early stage.
- A good time to do this is in or immediately after a bath or shower, when the muscles in the scrotum are relaxed.
- Partners may help with this.
- Hold the scrotum in the palms of the hands, so that the fingers and thumbs on both hands can be used to examine the testicles.
- Note the size and weight of the testicles.
- It is normal to have one testicle that is slightly larger and hangs lower than the other, but a noticeable change in weight or size may indicate that there is something wrong.
- Gently feel each testicle individually. It should feel smooth, with no swellings or lumps.
- It is unusual to develop cancer in both testicles at the same time, so in order to check whether one is feeling normal, compare it with the other.
- If any change is noticed (in particular a lump or swelling, usually on the front or side of the testicle), it should be discussed with a doctor as soon as possible.

SEXUAL MEDICINE

GENERAL PROBLEMS

Common sexual problems presenting to GPs are:

In women • Low sexual desire • vaginismus • orgasmic dysfunction.

In men • Low sexual desire • premature ejaculation • erectile dysfunction.

Other sexual difficulties that may present include: • sexual variations, e.g. homosexuality, transexualism and sadomasochism • sexual abuse • rape.

Most sexual problems require a similar basic approach.

Diagnosis

History Ask about:
- The exact nature of the problem, e.g. related to libido, stimulation, intercourse or orgasm.
- The patient's and his or her partner's expectations.
- Intercourse, e.g.:
  - whether intercourse has ever been enjoyable
  - frequency, pain or difficulty
  - contraception.
- The present relationship and the partner's response to the problem. (Consider whether or not the partner has a sexual problem.)
- Family background and education.
- Previous sexual history.
- Religious/cultural beliefs.
- Medical history (e.g. endocrine disorders, alcohol and drugs).
- Obstetric history (e.g. infertility, terminations, stillbirth, postpartum depression, attitudes to breast-feeding).
- Present mental state (e.g. anxiety or depression).

Examination Physical examination is not always necessary, but can often play an important therapeutic role in reassuring the patient.

Investigations As appropriate, e.g. to exclude endocrine problems.

Management

Discussing sexual problems requires sensitivity and acceptance. An essential part of the consultation is permission-giving, allowing patients to discuss a subject that is often embarrassing and uncomfortable to them. Advice and provision of information may be all that is required.

Always consider referral for sex therapy (via Relate or local Family Planning Clinics).

LOW SEXUAL DESIRE

This is the most common sexual problem for which women seek help. Primary low sexual desire is often attributable to parental condemnation of sexuality during childhood or previous traumatic sexual experiences. Secondary low sexual desire is often related to relationship difficulties, specific events such as childbirth or depression, hormonal changes or other co-existing sexual problems. Underlying psychological problems are frequent, and specialist help is often required.

DYSPAREUNIA

Diagnosis

History Ask about the nature of the pain.
    If the pain is localised to the entrance to the vagina it is usually related to:

- lack of lubrication
- vaginismus (severe spasm of the vaginal muscles)
- other vulval or vaginal causes, e.g. infections, menopausal atrophic vaginitis, episiotomy problems, vulvitis of unknown cause.

    If the pain occurs on deep penetration it is usually due to lack of arousal or pelvic pathology, e.g. endometriosis (see p. 41) or PID (see p. 44).

Management

- Explore fears and anxieties. Ignorance about sexual anatomy and physiology is still common.
- Vulval burning or pain may be psychogenic and it is important to explore this possibility if there is no other clear cause.
- For vaginismus, encourage the woman to examine herself with a finger, and when she is more confident, encourage her partner to do the same.
- Referral to a sex therapist is often appropriate.
- Referral to a gynaecologist should be arranged if an organic cause is suspected.

ERECTILE DYSFUNCTION

More than 50% of men with erectile dysfunction have a physiological problem. Psychological factors may exacerbate the problem, or may be primary.

Diagnosis

History Ask about the exact nature of the problem. A psychological problem is more likely if the impotence is situational, i.e. the man is able to get an erection in the early morning or through masturbation, but not with his partner. A physical cause is more likely if erections are partial.

Explore drug history, e.g. alcohol, beta blockers, tricyclic antidepressants and ACE inhibitors.

Examination Look for:
- Peripheral vascular disease, more likely in men with hypertension, a history of ischaemic heart disease or smokers. Check the femoral and peripheral pulses and measure blood pressure.
- Neurological signs, e.g. autonomic neuropathy.
- Signs of endocrine dysfunction. Examine the genitalia and secondary sexual characteristics.

Investigations Take blood for: ● fasting blood sugar ● testosterone ● thyroid function tests ● prolactin ● LH and FSH.

Management
- Refer for psychosexual counselling if appropriate.
- Treatment with sildenafil (Viagra) is usually effective, irrespective of the cause, at a starting dose of 50 mg (25 mg in the elderly) approximately 1 hour before sexual activity. It should not be used in those receiving nitrates. The guidelines for NHS prescribing are very specific; most patients will need private prescriptions.
- Consider referral to a urologist, e.g. for vasoactive injections, penile prostheses or vacuum devices.

PREMATURE EJACULATION

This is very common, particularly in young men having their first sexual relationships. It can usually be treated satisfactorily by the stop/start or the squeeze technique: when the man feels close to ejaculation he should stop and relax for 30 seconds, or the woman should squeeze the glans for 30 seconds. Stimulation can then continue and the process may be repeated. The man will eventually improve his control. Referral for psychosexual counselling is often appropriate.

ORGASMIC PROBLEMS

A woman with primary anorgasmia should be encouraged to experiment with her own sexual responses by masturbation or vibrator. Clitoral stimulation can then be incorporated into normal love-making. Consider referral for psychosexual counselling.

PAEDIATRICS

EXAMINATION OF THE NEONATE

Examination of the neonate should be completed and recorded at all deliveries within 24 hours of the birth. One in 40 newborns will be found to have a congenital malformation. The aim is to assess the baby's general condition and respiratory function, and to identify any special management requirements in the first few days.

Routine examination should include:

- *Measurements*: check weight and head circumference.
- *General appearance*: look for dysmorphic features. Assess general muscle tone. Jaundice appearing within 24 hours requires urgent attention.
- *Head*: look for abnormalities in the cranial shape, allowing for moulding. An unusually full anterior fontanelle suggests hydrocephalus and an ultrasound should be arranged.
- *Eyes*: look for eye-size asymmetry. (Discrepancy suggests an infection, a developmental defect, or congenital glaucoma, which is an emergency.) Look for the red reflex to exclude a cataract.
- *Nose*: look for signs of obstruction.
- *Mouth*: check the palate for clefts.
- *Chest*: observe respiratory movements. Auscultate, if appropriate.
- *Heart*: heart murmurs are common at birth. Checking for murmurs at 8 weeks is more selective.
- *Abdomen*: look for distension or organomegaly. Exclude a single umbilical artery.
- *Groins*: check femoral pulses which may be absent in aortic coarctation. Look for hernias.
- *Genitalia*: check that the testes are in the scrotum. Exclude hypospadias and epispadias, and sexual ambiguity.
- *Anus*: exclude imperforate anus. The passing of meconium excludes this.
- *Spine*: exclude a scoliosis. Exclude any possible spinal cord abnormalities by looking for naevi, lumps, pits or hairy patches over the spine.
- *Hips*: exclude congenital dislocation.

6–8-WEEK CHECK

This check is completed by the GP and is combined with the first immunisations. It should include:

- *Discussion of parental concerns*: ask about vision, hearing and general development. Ask how the parents and siblings are adjusting to the birth of the baby.

- *General observation*: look for alertness, response to handling, dysmorphic features, etc.
- *Skin*: ask about and look for blemishes and abnormalities.
- *Growth*: plot weight, head circumference and, where necessary, length on a centile chart.
- *Eyes*: look for abnormal movements, squint or failure of fixation.
- *Heart*: check for murmurs.
- *Genitalia*: check that the testes are in the scrotum. Exclude hypospadias and epispadias, and sexual ambiguity.
- *Hips*: exclude congenital dislocation.

ROUTINE CHILDHOOD VACCINATIONS

See page 194.

All newborn babies should receive vitamin K to prevent vitamin K deficiency bleeding (haemorrhagic disease of the newborn). Some areas recommend a single intramuscular vitamin K injection at birth. Other areas recommend oral vitamin K, two doses to be given in the first week of life (usually by the midwife). Babies who are being >50% breast-fed should receive a third oral dose at age 4 weeks (usually given by the health visitor).

NEONATAL JAUNDICE

- Jaundice within 24 hours of birth is always pathological.
- Serum bilirubin should be checked in babies with significant jaundice. Refer if the level lies above the limit for the baby's age. (Discuss with laboratory.)
- 'Physiological' jaundice appears after 48 hours and usually disappears by day 7–10 of life.
- Jaundice persisting or presenting after 10 days of age (14 days in immature babies) is abnormal and the baby should be referred for assessment. If the prolonged jaundice is associated with breast-feeding it should fade by 6 weeks of age.

INFANT FEEDING

BREAST-FEEDING

See page 35.

BOTTLE-FEEDING

Bottle-fed babies, like breast-fed babies, should be fed on demand and allowed to find their own pattern. Formula milk, as opposed to cow's milk (which has relatively low iron and vitamin A, C, D and E content), should ideally be given until the baby is 1 year old. The baby requires about 150 ml per kg body weight per day. This is usually given as about six feeds/bottles per day. In the first week or so, the baby takes about 50–70 ml 7–8 times per day.

Formula milks There are two groups of formula milk:
1. whey-based (with a whey/casein ratio similar to human milk)
2. casein-based (with the whey/casein ratio of cow's milk).

Whey-based formulae are generally recommended. The casein-based formulae are promoted on the basis that they are more satisfying. Changing milks because the baby has colic or seems unsettled is of no value. Soya milks are often misused. They have no advantage over other formulae but should be reserved for proven cow's milk intolerance.

Milk feeds after 6 months
● Formula milk should ideally be continued for the first year.
● Cow's milk can be introduced after 6 months.
● Low-fat milk should not be introduced before the age of 2.

WEANING

Weaning is the transition from an all-milk diet to a varied diet using solid foods. Advice should be sought from the health visitor.

● Solid foods are usually introduced by 6 months, but not before 3 months.
● Food should be offered by spoon in small quantities. If a food is rejected, it should be tried again after a while.
● Early foods should be low in salt and sugar.
● Plain rice cereals mixed with milk are usually given first, followed by stewed and puréed fruit or vegetables.
● As the baby starts to cut down milk consumption, small quantities of protein foods, e.g. meat or fish, can be added.
● By 9–12 months infants should be encouraged to have three regular meals per day, eating normal chopped family food. They will need about 0.5 litre (1 pint) of milk (breast, formula or cow's) per day, as well as additional fluids. Only give drinks after meals, to avoid reducing appetite. Water should be encouraged, and fruit juices should be diluted with water.
● Avoid an excessively high fibre intake, as high-fibre foods are bulky and have a relatively low nutrient and energy content.

- Supplementary vitamins (A, D and C), 5 drops daily from 6 months to 5 years, may be given to children with an inadequate diet.
- If, from the age of 6 months, a child uses fluoride toothpaste, fluoride supplements (even in areas where there is no added fluoride in the water supply) are now considered unnecessary.

BABIES WITH COLIC

When called to see a crying baby, important physical causes must be excluded, e.g. volvulus, intussusception or acute infection (e.g. otitis media or UTI).

Colic tends to start after 2 weeks of age, and usually settles by 4 months of age. The infant is often well in the morning, but by the evening may be distraught, pale and drawing up its legs. The parents are often quite unable to comfort the baby. They need reassurance that the problem is self-limiting and that they are not at fault since there is no clear cause. Involve the health visitor and encourage the parents to get as much rest as possible. Changing milk formulae is rarely helpful. Breast-feeding technique may need attention. A consistent feeding and sleeping routine may help, as may increased carrying and treatment with e.g. dimethicone (Infacol) 0.5–1 ml before feeds. Be alert for a child at risk (see child protection, p. 93).

Crying for long periods of time, especially in the evening, is usually due to 'colic'.

CONSTIPATION

CONSTIPATION IN INFANTS

Constipation is more common in formula-fed than in breast-fed babies. It is only considered to be a problem if hard stools cause straining and discomfort. The passage of a normal soft stool once a week, for example, is not a problem. The cause is not always clear, but it may be due to inadequate fluid intake or to inadequately diluted artificial feeds.

Management
- Consider the possibility of Hirschsprung's disease if there is delay in first passing meconium and subsequent constipation.
- Exclude an anal fissure.

- Encourage the parent to give abundant fluids. (Unsweetened fruit juice can be given to babies in addition to milk.)
- Abdominal massage can be helpful.
- Laxatives are very rarely required.

CONSTIPATION AND SOILING IN OLDER CHILDREN

Hard stools may cause faecal retention and chronic constipation. This can lead to soiling due to a distended rectum, which leads to relaxation of the internal sphincter. The external sphincter is then put under considerable strain and is unable to prevent leakage of faeces. Most children are clean by 2.5 years of age and soiling may be viewed as abnormal after 4 years of age.

Acute constipation often follows febrile illnesses.

Diagnosis

History Ask about: • the child's diet and fluid intake • previous bowel habit • present management and how the parents are coping.

Examination Check: • the abdomen for a loaded colon • the anus for an anal fissure • the rectum for the presence of faeces.

Management
The aim of treatment is to regain the child's confidence in being able to defaecate painlessly.

- An enema may be required to dislodge a faecal mass. However, this can be distressing for a child, and a course of an oral stimulant laxative is an alternative treatment, e.g. senna syrup (age >6 years, 5–10 ml in the morning). A short course of e.g. lactulose solution (age 5–10 years, 10 ml b.d.) is usually sufficient in cases of acute constipation.
- Encourage copious fluids and a high-fibre diet.
- Refractory cases may require a prolonged course of senna and/or lactulose in gradually reducing dosage in order to amplify the gastrocolic reflex. Consider referral to a paediatric gastroenterology clinic.
- The child should be encouraged to go to the toilet after each meal in order to encourage the gastrocolic reflex. Ensure that the child has sufficient, unhurried time to go to the toilet.
- The child with intentional defaecation in unacceptable places (encopresis) should be referred to a child psychiatrist.

NOCTURNAL ENURESIS

Bed-wetting in children is a common problem. Most children are dry at night by the age of 3, 90% are dry by the age of 5 and >95% by the age of 10. The cause of bed-wetting is usually unclear, but about 1% of children will have an organic problem, e.g. a congenital abnormality of the urinary tract, a urinary tract infection, polyuria or a neuropathic bladder.

Diagnosis

History Ask about:

- Whether the child has ever been dry. (A period of dryness suggests that the problem is not organic unless the child has an acute UTI.)
- Whether the child wets during the day. (After the age of 4 this suggests a neuropathic bladder and the child should be referred.)
- Family history. Children often follow a familial pattern.
- Any behavioural or emotional problems.
- Heavy sleeping.

Investigations • Dipstick urine for glucose, nitrite, leucocytes and protein • send urine for culture.

Management

Involve both the parent and the child, as well as the health visitor. Some areas have specific enuresis clinics.

> Specific treatment is unnecessary under the age of 7 years. Ten per cent of 5-year-olds still wet the bed.

Advice

- Drinks should be avoided in the evening.
- Lifting the child to the lavatory when the parent goes to bed may be helpful.
- A star chart with stars given for dry beds encourages the child.
- A child who is <7 years of age should wear nappies or trainer pants at night if the above methods are unsuccessful.

Treatment An enuresis alarm can be used if the above methods fail (obtainable via health visitors, school nurses or the local enuresis clinic). This is placed in the child's bed so that the alarm rings when the child wets. Most children become dry within 2–3 months. Stop using the alarm after about 28 consecutive dry nights. Relapse responds well to re-treatment.

Drug treatment is usually helpful in children who do not respond to conservative measures. Treatment is usually for a period of 3 months. A further course may be started after reassessment. Use e.g. desmopressin nasal spray (synthetic analogue of ADH) 20–40 μg at bedtime, or imipramine 25–75 mg at bedtime. Desmopressin can be used intermittently, e.g. when staying away from home. Imipramine has a high frequency of adverse effects and should be used with caution.

Refer to a urologist if history, examination or investigations suggest an organic cause, or if response to treatment is poor.

> A child with a neuropathic bladder has daytime as well as night-time wetting. Examine for absent ankle jerks and a sacral dimple or hairy naevus. Refer to a urologist.

URINARY TRACT INFECTION IN CHILDREN

(See also UTI, p. 64.)

Eight per cent of girls and 2% of boys will have a UTI in childhood. From 25% to 50% of children with UTIs have associated urinary tract abnormalities (mainly vesicoureteric reflux). Appropriate and prompt antibiotic treatment reduces the risk of renal damage, which can occur in children as a result of recurrent UTIs.

Consider a UTI in any child who is failing to thrive or who has symptoms of fever, vomiting, diarrhoea or irritability. Initial treatment of a suspected UTI is with antibiotics, e.g. trimethoprim or nitrofurantoin (see BNF for dose according to age) for 7 days, analgesia, if appropriate, and copious fluids.

Management
Follow local guidelines if available:

> ⚠ **All children under 5 years of age with a first confirmed UTI should be referred to a paediatric urologist for further investigation (e.g. ultrasound, micturating DMSA scan, cystogram). Arrange an ultrasound while awaiting specialist assessment.**

- Children over 5 years of age should have an ultrasound of the kidneys, ureters and bladder, including post-voiding residual urine volume, and should be referred to a paediatric urologist if this is abnormal.
- Antibiotic treatment should not be delayed while awaiting results of microscopy or culture.
- Antibiotic prophylaxis should be given to under 3 year olds, and to older children where there is likely to be delay before investigation, e.g. trimethoprim 1–2 mg/kg at night or nitrofurantoin 1 mg/kg at night. Antibiotic prophylaxis should also be considered for children with recurrent UTIs who have already been investigated.

- Arrange a repeat urine for microscopy and culture 1 month after the UTI, to ensure resolution.

SLEEP PROBLEMS

Sleep problems are very common and are nearly always simply habitual. Parents may be concerned that the child will not go to sleep, wakes during the night, or wakes very early. They are likely to be exhausted, and will need reassurance. Try to involve *both* parents in consistent management. Always consider involving the health visitor.

Exclude specific problems, e.g. unhappiness, fear, bed-wetting, environmental noise or illness.

Management

Advice

- An initial sleep diary, recording details of the sleep disturbance, is extremely useful. It should include waking time in the morning, times and lengths of naps during the day, time that the child went to bed, time of settling in bed, and times and lengths of waking during the evening and night, as well as parent management.
- Instil a disciplined bedtime routine.
- If the child gets out of bed, put him or her straight back with a firm reminder that it is time to sleep. Unless this plan is adhered to every time without fail, the child will continue to wake in the knowledge that the parent will eventually give way.
- Avoid rewards for night-waking, e.g. drinks, taking the child to the parents' bed.
- Ensure a satisfactory environment, e.g. night light, adequate warmth.
- As far as possible, reward success and avoid chastisement.
- Consider the short-term use of hypnotics, in addition to the above, especially if parents are experiencing difficulty coping, e.g. promethazine 15–20 mg (2–5 years), 20–25 mg (5–10 years), at bedtime.

NAPPY RASH

Nappy rash is nearly always either due to contact with ammonia from urine or due to *Candida* (thrush).

Management

- Change nappies frequently to avoid prolonged contact with urine.

- Encourage periods without a nappy, i.e. exposure of buttocks to air.
- Wash the nappy area with water at each change.
- Apply a barrier cream at each nappy change, e.g. zinc and castor oil cream.
- Regular use of bath oils and moisturising creams prevents skin dryness.

Candidal dermatitis usually presents as erythematous spots with satellite lesions, and often affects the flexures. (Ammoniacal dermatitis tends to spare the flexures.) Use an imidazole cream or nystatin cream ± a steroid cream, e.g. Timodine.

PRESCHOOL CHECK

This check is carried out by the GP when the child is 3.5 years old. The aim is to detect any potential special educational needs, as well as physical and emotional problems, and arrange for referral and assessment where necessary.

- Discuss parental concerns, asking specifically about vision, hearing, language and behaviour.
- Growth: plot height and weight on a centile chart.
- Examine heart and testes.
- Further examination is only necessary if indicated by parental concerns.
- Immunisations (see p. 194).

GROWTH PROBLEMS

Growth reflects general health and also the nutritional and emotional environment of a child. (For standard growth charts for girls and boys see appendices, pp. 376–379.)

Regular weight and head circumference measurements are useful to detect abnormalities and to reassure the parents that the baby is thriving.

FAILURE TO THRIVE

If the infant's growth pattern is causing concern:

- Measure and plot the infant's weight and head circumference at 2-weekly intervals and plot all previous measurements.
- Discuss milk intake, diet, nature and frequency of stools, and parental attitude and concerns.
- Perform a full examination.
- Check urine for protein, nitrite and leucocytes and send for culture.

- Discuss with the health visitor and other members of the primary healthcare team who may be involved.
- Refer if concern persists.

The most common reason for poor weight gain in breast-fed babies is insufficient milk intake. After attention to feeding technique, a trial of complementary bottle-feeding should be considered.

> Serious abnormalities affecting growth, in addition to poor weight gain, are usually accompanied by other symptoms and signs. Most babies who gradually cross centiles downwards are normal and are simply adopting their true growth trajectory.

FAT BABIES

Babies whose weight lies above the 97th centile should only be a cause for concern in extreme cases. Infant obesity is not a good predictor of adult obesity.

HEAD GROWTH

Large head
The most common cause of head enlargement is a familial large head, where the head circumference may cross centiles upwards, but additional symptoms are absent. Hydrocephalus usually presents as a head measurement that is crossing centile lines upwards, together with signs of raised intracranial pressure (e.g. tense fontanelle, suture separation, irritability).

- Measure the parents' head circumferences.
- Examine the baby for signs of raised intracranial pressure.
- Refer if there is concern.

Small head
Refer if the head circumference is below the 3rd centile.

SHORT/TALL STATURE

Short stature is considered to be a height below the 3rd centile, tall stature is above the 97th centile (see pp. 380–383). Both are usually normal variants. If there is concern about a child's height:

- Plot the child's height and weight together with previous recordings.
- To assess the expected final adult height of the child, plot the mean parental centile at age 19 (adult) on the growth chart:

– for a boy this is [father's height + (mother's height + 12.5 cm)]/2
– for a girl this is [father's height + (mother's height – 12.5 cm)]/2.

A height 8.5 cm above the mean centile is the 97th centile; 8.5 cm below it is the 3rd centile.

If the child's predicted final adult height is reasonably consistent with the mean parental centile, monitor the height. Refer if this is not the case, if centile lines are crossed or if there is concern about predicted final height.

RESPIRATORY PROBLEMS

CORYZA

There is rarely any need for antibiotic treatment. Consider paracetamol syrup to reduce irritability, and nasal decongestants if feeding is difficult, e.g. xylometazoline paediatric nasal drops, 2 drops per nostril t.d.s. (maximum duration of use 7 days).

COUGH

Bronchiolitis
Bronchiolitis usually presents as an irritable cough with tachypnoea after coryzal symptoms in infants and toddlers. There may be feeding difficulty and a low-grade fever. The most common cause is respiratory syncitial virus. Examination confirms widespread crepitations, especially on expiration. Advise provision of warm moist air, if appropriate. Confident supportive care of the child is important. Refer if there is significant feeding difficulty or if the child is ill. Antibiotics do not help.

Croup
Croup involves fever, rhinorrhoea and sore throat, together with the diagnostic features of inspiratory stridor and a barking cough. Calm, confident management is important. Ask the parents to place the child in a steamy room (e.g. boil the kettle without a lid), and the symptoms will often improve after 10–20 minutes. Antibiotics do not help. Refer if there is intercostal recession or if the child is ill. Before transfer to hospital, consider giving a single dose of oral dexamethasone 150 µg/kg or nebulised budesonide 2 mg.

Whooping cough (pertussis)
See page 180.

ASTHMA IN CHILDREN UNDER 5 YEARS OF AGE
See also page 164.

There is no evidence that early diagnosis or treatment affects the long-term prognosis of asthma in children under age 5.

Acute viral wheezy episodes in very young children are probably clinically distinct from atopic asthma.

The diagnosis of asthma in young children relies almost entirely on history.

History Ask about:
- a persistent nocturnal cough (a very common presentation in young children)
- recurrent wheezing (most commonly induced by exercise, upper respiratory tract infections and allergens).

Investigations Consider a chest X-ray if e.g. the child has recurrent chest infections or there is poor response to treatment.

Management of chronic asthma
- Avoid provoking factors, where appropriate. (Parents who smoke should be strongly advised against it.)
- Consider the best method of drug delivery:
  – Age 0–2: MDI + spacer and face mask. Bronchodilator syrups, e.g. salbutamol syrup 100 µg/kg t.d.s. p.r.n. (unlicensed at this age), have more systemic side-effects and are less effective, but are frequently used in mild cases or for diagnostic treatment trials.
  – Age 3–5: MDI + spacer.
  Nebulisers are rarely needed. Spacer devices are cheaper and as effective.
- Involve parents in a self-management plan as far as possible.
- Regularly review compliance, inhaler technique and parental concerns, especially before stepping treatment up or down.

Drug therapy Start the patient at the appropriate step according to symptoms.

Step 1 Occasional use of relief bronchodilators as required, e.g. salbutamol 200 µg (2 puffs).

Step 2 In addition to step 1, start either cromoglycate via MDI + spacer 10 mg t.d.s. *or* an inhaled steroid, e.g. beclomethasone up to 400 µg daily or fluticasone up to 200 µg daily.

Step 3 Refer to a paediatrician for consideration of:
- increasing the inhaled steroid
- adding a long-acting β agonist (e.g. salmeterol) or a slow-release xanthine
- oral steroids.

A 5-day course of soluble prednisolone (<1 year, 1–2 mg/kg/day; 1–5 years, 20 mg/day) should be considered at any time to gain rapid control.

Management of acute asthma   See page 167.

CONVULSIONS

NON-FEBRILE CONVULSIONS

Diagnosis

History Ask about: ● loss of consciousness ● shaking or jerking ● incontinence ● post-ictal state ● period of amnesia ● family history.

General management
- Admit all infants with a convulsion under the age of 6 months.
- Refer older children who have had a convulsion to a paediatric neurology clinic.
- Children with epilepsy should not cycle in traffic. They may swim in the presence of a responsible adult.
- The tendency to have seizures resolves during childhood in >60% of children. Anticonvulsant therapy can be stopped, on specialist advice, if the child has been free from seizures for 2 or 3 years.

Management of status epilepticus
- Ensure that the airway is patent.
- Give diazepam 0.3 mg/kg i.v. slowly, or rectally 2.5 mg (age <1), 5 mg (age 1–3), 10 mg (age >3).
- Admit the child if fitting continues.

FEBRILE CONVULSIONS

Febrile convulsions are very common, affecting about 4% of all children, usually in the second year of life.

Diagnosis

History The child has usually been unwell with a high fever when he or she develops a major motor seizure lasting a few minutes. There is often a family history of febrile convulsions.

Examination
- The child has a fever and often an upper respiratory tract infection.
- Look for signs of meningitis.

- Examine ears and throat.
- Examine the chest.
- Examine the abdomen.

Investigations Send a urine sample for culture, if appropriate.

Management
Admit if:

1. meningitis is suspected
2. the child is <18 months old
3. the fit lasts for more than 10 minutes
4. the child is clearly unwell
5. there are persistent neurological signs
6. more than one fit occurs during one febrile episode.

The child may be left at home if the fit lasts for <10 minutes and recovery is complete.

The risk of recurrence after one febrile convulsion is about 20%. This may be minimised by advising the parents to use tepid sponging and paracetamol whenever the child becomes febrile.

Paracetamol doses: age 3 months to 1 year, 60–120 mg, 4–6 hourly p.r.n.; age 1–5 years, 120–250 mg, 4–6 hourly p.r.n.; age 6–12 years, 250–500 mg, 4–6 hourly p.r.n. (maximum of four doses in 24 hours).

CHILD PROTECTION

Child abuse is often divided into four categories. Few actual cases in practice fall neatly into one category.

1. PHYSICAL ABUSE

Physical abuse should be suspected where the nature of the injury is not consistent with the account of how it occurred, *or* where there is reasonable suspicion that the injury was inflicted or knowingly not prevented. There is often delay in seeking medical attention. Suspicious injuries include:
• handslap marks • facial and neck bruising • bruising to soft body parts, e.g. buttocks, lower abdomen or thighs • cigarette burns • grip marks • bite marks • 'dipping' scalds • torn frenulum.
Physical abuse includes Munchausen syndrome by proxy.

2. SEXUAL ABUSE

This includes direct and indirect (e.g. pornography and indecent exposure) sexual acts perpetrated on a child who is either too young to give consent, or is old enough to give consent but is in an exploitative relationship.

Examination is usually unhelpful, but there may be genital or anal injury, emotional disturbance or sexually inappropriate behaviour. The most common presentation is with a statement by the child or by another member of the family.

3. NEGLECT

This involves persistent neglect and failure to protect the child from exposure to danger or threats to health. It may present as failure to thrive, severe nappy rash, unkempt condition, developmental delay or behavioural and emotional disturbance.

4. EMOTIONAL ABUSE

This involves severe psychological mistreatment. The child is denied comfort, nurture, control and love. There may be persistent verbal denigration and humiliation in the absence of positive interest.

CHILD PROTECTION PROCEDURES

 The child's welfare is paramount. The duty of confidentiality is overridden by the duty to protect the child from abuse.

Children's best interests are served by being cared for within their own families wherever this is possible.

- Take a full history, and carefully record observations.
- Fully examine the child, except in cases of possible sexual abuse when examination should be carried out only by doctors with appropriate training.
- Expert anonymous consultative advice is always available in doubtful cases from e.g. child protection coordinators at Social Services.
- Discuss with other appropriate members of the Primary Healthcare Team, particularly the health visitor.

    If abuse is suspected:

- Refer as soon as possible to the Child Protection Investigation Team at Social Services. They will consider the need to remove the child to a place of safety.

- Refer for further medical examination:
  - for physical abuse, to the paediatric registrar on-call (immediately)
  - for sexual abuse, to an approved doctor
  - for neglect or emotional abuse, to a paediatric consultant.

The degree of urgency depends on the severity and type of abuse, the age of the child (younger children are more vulnerable), and continued exposure to risk.

- Involve the parents as far as is possible.
- Attend the case conference, or provide a written report. The child may be placed on the Child Protection Register for regular monitoring.
- The case may be taken to court where a supervision order or a care order may be issued.

SUDDEN INFANT DEATH

Sudden infant death syndrome (SIDS) is defined as the sudden, unexpected death of an infant or young child, for which post-mortem fails to show a cause. It occurs in one in 500 live births and there is a peak incidence between 2 and 3 months of age. It is rare after 6 months.

Management
The management of families suffering a sudden infant death has similarities with other cases of bereavement (see p. 333).

A phone call from parents whose baby has stopped breathing
- Call an ambulance if the parents have not done so.
- Tell the parents you will come immediately.
- Has resuscitation been attempted? Tell the parents how to attempt mouth-to-mouth resuscitation.
- Continue resuscitation until the ambulance arrives, unless the child is clearly dead (see below).

The 'near miss' (i.e. the apnoeic child has been resuscitated) Admit the child to hospital. The risk of further episodes or of sequelae, whether real or perceived, is lessened by hospital admission.

The dead baby

Immediate action
- Confirm death (see p. 331).
- Comfort parents and siblings. Be prepared for severe grief reactions, including anger.
- Try to answer parents' questions, which often reflect their feelings of guilt.

- Inform the coroner, who will arrange for the baby to be taken to a mortuary. Usually a uniformed policeman or woman will be sent to take a statement from the parents.
- Encourage the parents to hold their dead baby.
- Suggest the parents call a close friend or family member to help. This also allows the GP to leave.

Later action
- Visit the family soon after the death.
- Listen to parents' and siblings' expressions of grief.

Common features of grief
These include guilt, anger, loss of confidence, fear of being alone and a sense of unfairness. Many parents have vivid dreams and hear the baby crying.

- Painful, engorged breasts due to the sudden cessation of breast-feeding can be relieved by bromocriptine tab. 2.5 mg daily for 3 days, increased to twice daily if necessary for up to 2 weeks.
- Involve others in support, e.g.:
  - health visitor or midwife
  - Cot Death Helpline (Foundation for the Study of Infant Deaths) (see p. 385).
- Offer referral to a paediatrician for the parents to discuss the death.
- Offer continued support at home, in the surgery or over the telephone.

Parents' anxieties over the next pregnancy and baby following a sudden infant death
- Common feelings are doubt, loss of confidence, and fear of loving the new baby too much.
- Reassure the parents that the risk of further SIDS is very low and involve others in supporting the family, e.g. health visitor and midwife, paediatrician and CONI (Care of Next Infant) (see p. 385).
- Apnoea monitors, room thermometers, weighing scales and charts are available from the Foundation for the Study of Infant Deaths (see p. 385).
- Offer same-day appointments for minor illnesses.

Primary prevention of sudden infant death Advise all pregnant women and mothers of babies to avoid:

- overwrapping the baby in the cot
- placing the baby face down to sleep
- smoking.

ENDOCRINOLOGY

DIABETES

A GP with a list of 2000 patients might expect to have 50 patients with diabetes, 10–15 of whom will be receiving insulin at any one time.

Many people with diabetes, particularly those with type 2 ('non-insulin-dependent diabetes mellitus' or NIDDM) remain undiagnosed for years and may present with advanced retinopathy, neuropathy or macrovascular disease.

All pregnant women should be screened for diabetes.

> Active case-finding and organised screening of selected groups is the key to diagnosis.

Risk factors in diabetes
The following factors put people at increased risk of developing diabetes:

- >65 years old
- Asian or Afro-Caribbean origin
- obesity, particularly abdominal obesity
- a family history of diabetes or cardiovascular disease
- a history of gestational diabetes
- a history of having delivered a large baby (>4.5 kg) ⎫ in women.
- a history of unexplained foetal loss ⎭

Diagnosis

History Patients with the following symptoms should be tested for diabetes:
- thirst, polyuria and weight loss
- recurrent infections, especially skin infections
- neuropathic symptoms, e.g. pain, numbness and paraesthesiae
- marked visual acuity changes
- unexplained symptoms, e.g. lassitude.

> Diabetes is defined by WHO criteria, using venous samples, as:
>
> - a fasting blood glucose level of >7 mmol/l, or
> - a random plasma glucose level of >11.1 mmol/l.
>
> In asymptomatic patients the measurements should be duplicated on another day before the diagnosis is made.

Investigations

Patients with a fasting plasma glucose between 6.1 and 7.0 mmol/l have impaired fasting glycaemia and need an oral glucose tolerance test to exclude diabetes, and annual follow-up. (See WHO criteria, p. 98.)

The oral glucose tolerance test
- The patient should not have smoked and should have had a normal carbohydrate intake for the previous 3 days.
  - After an overnight fast, give 75 g of oral glucose (350 ml of Lucozade can be used).
  - Measure blood glucose 2 hours later.
- Diabetes is defined as a 2-hour plasma glucose level of >11.1 mmol/l.

Management

Referral At the time of diagnosis, if the patient is ill, ketonuria is present, or if the blood glucose is more than about 25 mmol/l, immediate referral should be arranged.

Admit all children and pregnant women.

Aims of diabetic care
- To keep the patient well and symptom-free.
- To keep the fasting blood glucose below 6.7 mmol/l, the maximum blood glucose below 10 mmol/l and the level 2 hours after a meal below 6.7 mmol/l. (It is generally believed that good diabetic control prevents the development of long-term complications.)
- To avoid fasting glycosuria.
- To maintain the HbA_{1c} below 7%.
- To minimise the risk of cardiovascular disease by vigorously treating hypertension and hypercholesterolaemia in conjunction with the diabetes. All diabetics should be prescribed aspirin 75 mg o.d. and a statin, e.g. simvastatin 10–20 mg o.d.
- To detect complications early, in order to reduce:
  - angina, MI and cerebrovascular disease
  - foot ulceration and limb amputation due to peripheral vascular disease and diabetic neuropathy
  - visual loss due to diabetic retinopathy
  - renal failure due to diabetic nephropathy.
- To offer effective education.

General management

Practice nurses and diabetes specialist nurses have a valuable role in sharing the management of the diabetic patient. Diabetes UK is the national association for diabetes (see p. 385) and offers excellent on-line advice to both patients and professionals.

Education
- Emphasise the importance of self-management.
- Advise against smoking.
- Self-monitoring:
  - All type 1 (insulin-dependent diabetes mellitus (IDDM)) patients should measure their blood glucose (and, ideally, their urine for ketonuria). Teach home glucose monitoring using a blood glucose test meter. Testing should ideally be carried out before each main meal and before bed.
  - Urine testing alone is satisfactory for older type 2 diabetics. The urine should be tested 2 hours after a meal. A series of three tests on one day per week is more useful than once-daily testing.
- Intercurrent illness:

> ⚠ **Diabetes therapy (insulin or tablets) should never be reduced or omitted during intercurrent illness. Insulin-dependent diabetics usually require *more* insulin during intercurrent illness.**

  - Non-insulin-treated patients can occasionally become ketoacidotic during intercurrent illness and may require insulin therapy.
  - The frequency of self-monitoring should be increased.
  - Fluid intake should be increased.
  - Daily carbohydrate intake should be maintained, as liquid if necessary.
  - If the blood glucose is >13 mmol/l or the urine sugar is ≥2%, increase the insulin by 2–4 units per day until control is regained.
  - Admit if the patient is vomiting and unable to take liquid or carbohydrate, or is ketoacidotic or dehydrated.
- Give advice on foot care. Look out for problems, e.g. corns, ingrowing toenails, bunions, and refer to podiatry if appropriate.
- Discuss the warning signs of hypoglycaemia (unsteadiness, difficulty in concentration, headache and tremulousness).
- Driving: patients must notify the Driver and Vehicle Licensing Agency and their insurance company.
- Free prescriptions: patients receiving treatment with either tablets or insulin are exempt from paying prescription charges.
- Occupation: hazardous jobs are no longer an option for patients with type 1 diabetes mellitus, e.g. police, armed forces.

- Diet:
  - Refer all newly diagnosed patients for dietary advice (practice nurse or dietician).
  - Overweight patients need advice on calorie reduction. Consider drug treatment for obesity (see p. 105).

> The main dietary message for diabetics is to eat 'healthily'. At least half of the energy intake should be made up of complex, fibre-rich carbohydrates. Intake of refined carbohydrate, fat, alcohol and salt should be low.

- Encourage exercise and increased physical activity.

Routine review The patient should be checked at least 6-monthly (either by the GP or hospital diabetic clinic).
  Look at:

- The patient's own records of blood or urine testing (self-monitoring).
- Fasting blood sugar.
- Weight/BMI (and discuss diet).
- Urine for protein. If present, send an MSU for microscopy and culture, and check serum creatinine. If the proteinuria is heavy, measure the 24-hour urinary protein. If this is high, exclude causes other than diabetic nephropathy, improve diabetic control and treat even mild hypertension.
    If proteinuria is absent, the urine should be checked for microalbuminuria. If positive, the patient should be started on an ACE inhibitor to delay the onset of nephropathy, even if the blood pressure is normal.

  Check annually:

- BP. Aiming to reduce to below 130/80 ideally.
- Visual acuity.
- Fundi (dilate pupils with 1% tropicamide). Fundoscopy can be performed by an optometrist, or referral can be made for regular fundal photography. Annual screening for diabetic retinopathy can now be performed by accredited opticians throughout the UK.
- Bloods:
  - HbA$_{1c}$, aiming for a value of below 7% ideally
  - serum creatinine, to exclude renal failure
  - serum cholesterol, triglyceride and HDL, aiming to reduce total cholesterol to below 5.0 mmol/l (the recently published Heart Protection Study probably lowers this threshold) by the use of statins.
- Feet:
  - pulses
  - reflexes
  - vibration and pin-prick sensation
  - evidence of ulceration, etc.

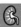

Therapeutic management of type 2 diabetes mellitus

> The primary treatment of type 2 diabetes is diet, with the aim of reducing excess weight and avoiding refined sugar.

Tablets and insulin should not be used before an adequate trial of diet and an increase in physical activity (2–3 months), unless the patient is very ill or has a very high blood glucose (>25 mmol/l).

For overweight patients, start with metformin, which decreases gluconeogenesis and increases peripheral utilisation of glucose, 500 mg b.d. (providing renal and hepatic function are normal) and increase the dose monthly as appropriate, to a maximum of 1 g b.d. Add a sulphonylurea (see below) if control remains inadequate.

For patients of normal weight, prescribe a sulphonylurea, which augments insulin secretion, e.g. gliclazide 40–80 mg daily, adjusted according to response up to a maximum of 160 mg. Warn the patient of the hazard of hypoglycaemia. Add metformin if control remains inadequate.

Other oral antidiabetic drugs include acarbose, nateglinide, repaglinide and the thiazolidinediones (see BNF).

If control remains poor despite attention to diet and tablets, insulin therapy should be considered.

Therapeutic management of type 1 diabetes mellitus Insulin doses are determined on an individual basis, by gradually increasing the dose but avoiding disabling hypoglycaemia. If the blood glucose is too high, increase the dose of insulin. If the blood glucose is too low, decrease it. Hypoglycaemia between 10 a.m. and lunchtime or between the evening meal and midnight is due to too much short-acting insulin in the morning or evening, respectively. Reduce the dose by 2–4 units.

Hypoglycaemia between 2 p.m. and the evening meal or during the night or before breakfast is due to too much long-acting insulin in the morning or evening, respectively. Reduce the dose by 4–6 units.

Hypoglycaemia Treat with oral glucose.

If the patient is unconscious, treat with 50% glucose 20–50 ml i.v., or glucagon 1 mg i.m., s.c. or i.v. (Glucagon can be issued to responsible relatives for emergency use.)

Prescription charge exemption Diabetics on oral antidiabetic drugs or insulin are exempt from prescription charges.

THYROID DISORDERS

HYPOTHYROIDISM

Hypothyroidism is common, especially in elderly people in whom the presenting signs are often non-specific. The threshold for testing should therefore be low.

Diagnosis

- Serum thyroid stimulating hormone (TSH) is the best initial screening test, as a normal value (0.05–6.0 mU/l) virtually excludes hypo- and hyperthyroidism.
- If the TSH is high, measure free T4. If this is low, hypothyroidism is confirmed.
- In subclinical hypothyroidism the TSH is high but the free T4 is normal, and when to start T4 replacement is a matter of clinical judgement.
- Problems with interpreting thyroid function tests in the elderly usually result from non-thyroidal illness or drug treatment.

Management

Most cases of hypothyroidism, particularly in the elderly, can be managed by the GP. Refer those who are young or ill. Check for autoantibodies (their presence makes other autoimmune diseases more likely).

Treatment Treat with oral thyroxine. The initial dose is 100 μg daily (50 μg for those >50 years) or 25–50 μg in elderly patients or those with cardiac disease. If the lower dose is started, increase the dose by 25 or 50 μg daily each month until 100 μg per day is reached.

Check the TSH each month and stop increasing the thyroxine dose when the TSH is normal. The usual maintenance dose of thyroxine is 100–200 μg daily. If the TSH is suppressed (<0.08 mU/l) in young people, the thyroxine dose should be lowered in order to avoid osteoporosis.

Follow-up Annual follow-up should be arranged. TFTs should be checked if under- or overtreatment is suspected (or in the young). Many authorities recommend annual testing. Serum TSH is the best single guide to T4 replacement therapy, as it provides a measure of thyroid function over the preceding weeks. The serum T4 level, however, changes more quickly than TSH, and it may be normal even if the patient has been non-compliant until just before sampling.

Prescription charge exemption Patients with hypothyroidism are exempt from prescription charges.

HYPERTHYROIDISM

Diagnosis

The best initial test is serum TSH. If this is suppressed, hyperthyroidism can be confirmed by a raised free T4. Free T3 levels should only be measured if the free T4 is normal, in order to make the diagnosis of T3 toxicosis which occurs in <5% of patients with hyperthyroidism.

Management

> Refer all patients for specialist assessment. The aetiology must be determined and the commonest causes are Graves' disease (80% of cases), toxic multinodular goitre and toxic adenoma.

While awaiting assessment, use propranolol 40 mg t.d.s. for rapid relief of symptoms if necessary, in conjunction with carbimazole.

Start carbimazole 15–40 mg daily and maintain the dose until the patient becomes euthyroid, usually after 4–8 weeks. Then reduce the dose progressively to a maintenance of 5–15 mg daily. Assess clinically and biochemically (serum T4) every 6 months. Carbimazole can rarely induce agranulocytosis, which may present as e.g. a sore throat. A white blood cell count should be performed if there is any clinical evidence of infection.

Carbimazole treatment is continued for 18 months in the hope of inducing life-long remission On stopping treatment, a combination of TSH and free T4 measurements is useful to assess thyroid status. Follow-up beyond 1 year is not necessary, but patients should be warned about the possible recurrence of symptoms.

THYROID ENLARGEMENT

A thyroid swelling can involve the whole gland (goitre) or consist of an isolated nodule.

> ⚠ **All thyroid nodules should be referred to a surgeon with a specialist interest, in order to exclude malignancy. A simple or multinodular goitre in a euthyroid patient need only be referred if it bothers the patient.**

OBESITY

Obesity is defined in terms of body mass index (BMI) (see p. 147):

- 25–30, overweight (grade I)
- 30–40, moderate obesity (grade II)
- >40, severe obesity (grade III).

About 30% of the UK population have grade I obesity, 3% have grade II obesity and 0.3% have grade III obesity. Mortality rates double at a BMI of 35, and increase exponentially with increasing BMI. Obesity is often associated with psychosocial problems, and can exacerbate various medical problems, including: • hypertension • ischaemic heart disease • diabetes mellitus • respiratory problems • arthritis • gallstones • varicose veins • intertrigo.

Management

- In order to lose weight, energy output must exceed energy input.
- Discuss breaking the diet/weight-gain/diet cycle by encouraging normal eating patterns.
- Think in the long term. Set realistic goals and take things slowly.
- The patient might expect to lose 0.5–1.0 kg per week on a reduced-calorie diet of e.g. 1000 kcal per day.
- In general, avoid the use of drugs for treating obesity, as they tend to work only in the short term. However, consider:
  - Orlistat 120 mg t.d.s. at mealtimes if the BMI is >30 or if the BMI is >28 in the presence of other risk factors, e.g. type 2 diabetes, hypertension, hypercholesterolaemia. It must be prescribed in the context of support, monitoring and counselling (see BNF guidelines).
  - Sibutramine 10–15 mg daily. Similar guidance to Orlistat license. BP must be checked regularly.
- Encourage regular exercise.
- Consider involving the practice nurse or hospital dietician. Outside agencies, e.g. Weight Watchers, can be very helpful.

GASTROENTEROLOGY

DYSPEPSIA

Dyspepsia covers a range of symptoms, including epigastric/oesophageal pain, fullness, early satiety, bloating and nausea. It accounts for 3–4% of GP consultations. The main causes are:

- non-ulcer or functional dyspepsia (60–70%)
- peptic ulcer disease (15–20%)
- gastro-oesophageal reflux disease (GORD) (5–15%)
- upper GI cancers (<2%) (less than 1 in 1 million under-55-year-olds with dyspepsia have cancer).

Diagnosis

History Ask about:
- aspects of the epigastric pain, e.g. relationship to food, periodicity, waking at night
- associated features, e.g. nausea and vomiting, changes in appetite, dietary indiscretion, alcohol intake, weight loss.

Alarm symptoms
Patients with dyspepsia who fulfil these criteria require referral for urgent endoscopy:

- dysphagia
- weight loss
- anaemia
- vomiting
- epigastric mass
- GI bleed.

Also:

- Age over 55 with onset of dyspepsia less than 1 year ago or continuous symptoms since onset.
- One of the following risk factors: family history of upper GI cancer in more than two first-degree relatives, Barrett's oesophagus, pernicious anaemia, peptic ulcer surgery over 20 years ago, known dysplasia, atrophic gastritis or intestinal metaplasia.

The following guidelines are for illustration only.

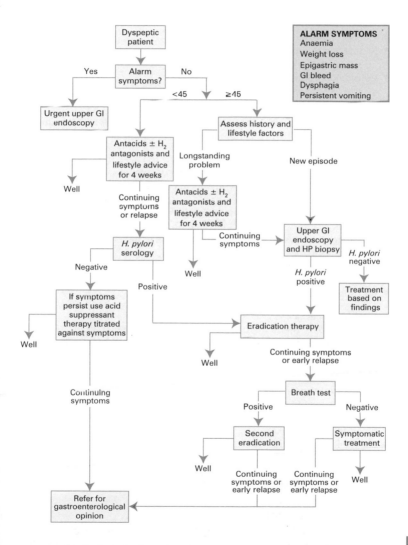

Oxfordshire Guidelines for the Management of Dyspepsia. Reproduced with permission of the Gastroenterology Unit, John Radcliffe Hospital, Oxford, UK

Management

Lifestyle advice
- Stop NSAIDs and aspirin.
- Stop smoking.
- Reduce coffee and alcohol intake.
- Lose weight, if appropriate.
- Consider stress factors.

Prescribing (See guidelines above for specific advice.)

Antacids/alginates: e.g. magnesium trisilicate 10 ml after meals and at bedtime, or p.r.n., or gaviscon 10–20 ml after meals and at bedtime or p.r.n.

Histamine H_2-receptor antagonists: e.g. cimetidine 400 mg b.d. for 4 weeks or ranitidine 150 mg b.d. for 4 weeks (see BNF for details).
   Low-dose maintenance treatment, e.g. cimetidine 400 mg nocte or ranitidine 150 mg nocte:
- largely replaced in *Helicobacter pylori* positive patients by eradication regimens
- in undiagnosed dyspepsia it may be acceptable in patients <45 only, but not long-term (see guidelines).
- for frequent severe recurrences
- for ulcer complications in the elderly
- for prophylactic use.

Proton pump inhibitors: e.g. lansoprazole 30 mg mane for 4 weeks:
- an effective short-term treatment for gastric and duodenal ulcers
- used in combination with antibacterials for *Helicobacter pylori* eradication.
- the treatment of choice for severe GORD or proven pathology, e.g. Barrett's oesophagus.

Low-dose maintenance treatment, e.g. lansoprazole 15 mg mane:
- do not use long-term without a confirmed diagnosis
- useful for severe GORD or for NSAID-associated ulceration where NSAID needs to be continued
- use the lowest dose for effective symptom relief.

Other treatments Symptoms of dysmotility, including nausea and bloating, may be treated with e.g. metoclopramide or domperidone.

HELICOBACTER PYLORI

H. pylori is associated with >90% of DUs, >80% of GUs and >60% of gastric cancers. It is not associated with GORD. Long-term healing of DUs and GUs can be achieved rapidly by eradicating *H. pylori*. Reinfection is rare. Confirm the presence of *H. pylori* before starting eradication treatment.

The presence of *H. pylori* should be confirmed before starting eradication treatment.

Tests for H. pylori

- Histology (endoscopic biopsy), breath tests and serology all have sensitivities and specificities >90%.
- Serology remains positive for up to 9 months after eradication.
- Breath tests (carbon–urea) become negative with *H. pylori* eradication, and are therefore used to confirm eradication, if appropriate. Breath test kits are prescribable on FP10.

H. pylori eradication

There are various eradication therapy regimens, e.g. lansoprazole 30 mg b.d. + amoxycillin 1 g b.d. + clarithromycin 500 mg b.d. for 7 days, or lansoprazole 30 mg b.d. + amoxycillin 1 g b.d. + metronidazole 400 mg b.d. for 7 days.

GASTRO-OESOPHAGEAL REFLUX DISEASE (GORD)

This is common. It usually presents as substernal pain, which is worse on lying flat, together with an acidic taste in the mouth. It is usually secondary to a hiatus hernia.

Management

Advice

- As for dyspepsia (see p. 108).
- Elevate the head of the bed.
- Avoid eating late in the evening.
- Avoid large meals.
- Lose any excess weight.
- Avoid foods which aggravate symptoms, e.g. fatty foods, alcohol, coffee, citrus fruits.

Prescribing (Prescribe according to severity.)

- Antacids (as for dyspepsia).
- Antiemetics and drugs which stimulate gastric emptying, e.g. metoclopramide or domperidone.
- High-dose H_2 receptor antagonists, e.g. cimetidine 400 mg b.d. or q.d.s. for 4–8 weeks, or ranitidine 150 mg b.d. or q.d.s. for 8–12 weeks. Maintenance treatment is cimetidine 400 mg o.d. or b.d., or ranitidine 150 mg o.d. or b.d.

Recurrent symptoms often require high-dose maintenance treatment. (Use the lowest dose for effective symptom relief.)

- Proton pump inhibitors, e.g. lansoprazole 30 mg daily for 4–8 weeks. Maintenance treatment is usually 15–30 mg daily. (Use the lowest dose for effective symptom relief.)

Referral Non-responders should be referred for a gastroenterological opinion.

HALITOSIS

When persistent, this is a distressing complaint and is usually due to poor oral hygiene or dental or gum sepsis.

Diagnosis

History Ask about:
- chronic sinusitis, tonsillitis, respiratory infections and mouth-breathing in children (adenoids)
- smoking and drugs, e.g. alcohol, isosorbide dinitrate, disulfiram
- dry mouth due to e.g. drugs, Sjögren's syndrome
- mood disorders which can present as halitosis.

Investigations These are rarely necessary, but it may be appropriate to exclude nasopharyngeal malignancy, upper GI tract pathology or metabolic disorders.

Management
- Refer to a dentist for oral assessment.
- Advise on oral hygiene.
- Use a mouth rinse, e.g. 0.2% aqueous chlorhexidine gluconate.

Antibiotic treatment is rarely necessary, but consider treatment with e.g. metronidazole or amoxycillin for 2 weeks to eradicate bacterial overgrowth.

INFECTIVE DIARRHOEA

Acute diarrhoea is usually due to food poisoning or a viral infection. Most patients recover spontaneously. Always consider alternative diagnoses, e.g. inflammatory bowel disease, drugs or ischaemic colitis.

Diagnosis

History Ask about: • ingestion of suspicious foods • any contacts with diarrhoea • occupation (food-handlers will require specific advice) • recent travel abroad • blood in the stools.

Investigations Send stool specimen for investigation if: ● diarrhoea is particularly severe ● diarrhoea has been present for >10 days ● there is blood in the stool ● there is a recent history of foreign travel ● the patient works with food.

Management

Advice
- Fluid intake should be copious.
- Food should not be withheld.
- Rehydration solutions may be helpful, especially in children (e.g. Dioralyte).
- On the whole antidiarrhoeal agents should be avoided, especially in children and the elderly.
- If necessary, diarrhoea in adults can be treated with e.g. loperamide two capsules stat. then one capsule after each loose stool.

Prescribing Indications for antibiotics are few, as they usually fail to influence the course of the illness and they can prolong and increase the frequency of the carrier state. Ciprofloxacin 500 mg b.d. for 5 days is occasionally used for prophylaxis against traveller's diarrhoea, but routine use is *not* recommended. Antibiotics are, however, indicated for:

- *Salmonella*, if severe (ciprofloxacin 500 mg b.d. for 5 days or trimethoprim 200 mg b.d. for 5 days).
- *Campylobacter* (erythromycin 500 mg q.d.s. for 5 days).
- *Giardiasis* (metronidazole 2 g daily for 3 days). Prompt response to antibiotic treatment is, in fact, a more reliable diagnostic test than stool examination in giardiasis, which is suspected with a >2-week incubation period, watery stools and excessive flatus without fever.
- *Shigella* (ciprofloxacin 500 mg b.d. for 5 days or trimethoprim 200 mg b.d. for 5 days).

Referral Refer if:
- there is dehydration
- there is toxaemia, abdominal pain or abdominal distension
- the diagnosis is unclear.

Administration
Notify, if appropriate (see notifiable diseases, p. 372).

PRURITUS ANI

A clear cause for pruritus ani is not always found. In children, the usual diagnosis is threadworms, especially if the history is short.

Diagnosis

History Attempt to exclude threadworms by asking about the presence of worms in the stools.

Ask about any perianal rash.

Examination Attempt to exclude the following:
- anorectal disease, e.g. haemorrhoids, fissures
- skin disease, e.g. psoriasis, contact dermatitis (including allergic reactions to products used to treat the pruritus)
- infection, e.g. fungal
- systemic disease, e.g. diabetes mellitus (fungal infection) and chronic liver disease.

Management

Threadworms Pruritus is due to perianal egg deposition. Examination is usually unnecessary. It is reasonable to treat only the affected child as long as the rest of the family are scrupulously attentive to hygiene. Alternatively, the whole family can be treated.

- Wash perianal skin each morning.
- Wash hands and nails after each visit to the lavatory.
- Treat with mebendazole 100 mg sachet stat. and repeat 2 weeks later if reinfection occurs, or piperazine powder one sachet stat. and repeat after 2 weeks.

General If no treatable cause is found:
- Consider treating empirically for threadworms.
- Advise careful perianal hygiene after defaecation with thorough drying.
- Avoid use of allergenic substances.
- Hydrocortisone ointment is useful, especially at night, or topical antifungal/ steroid mixtures.

ANAL FISSURE

See page 270.

CHANGE IN BOWEL HABIT

- Remember to perform a rectal examination.
- Check for anaemia and perform faecal occult bloods.
- Refer if the cause is unclear.

Suspect colonic carcinoma when a patient presents with unexplained, persistent change of bowel habit, either constipation or diarrhoea.

RECTAL BLEEDING

FRESH BLOOD

Fresh blood is usually the result of pathology between the anal margin and the lower sigmoid colon, e.g. haemorrhoids, anal fissure, diverticulitis, anorectal carcinoma.

- If the bleeding is minor in a patient aged <40 where the cause is clearly benign, e.g. haemorrhoids, it is reasonable to monitor symptoms over a period of time, and advise on avoiding constipation, etc.
- Remember to perform a rectal examination.
- Check Hb, if appropriate.

All patients aged >40, with new symptoms or where the bleeding is significant, or where there are associated symptoms, e.g. weight loss, change in bowel habit, should be referred for proctoscopy/sigmoidoscopy/barium enema, etc.

See also haemorrhoids (p. 270).

MELAENA OR ALTERED BLOOD

This suggests bleeding from further up the GI tract. Melaena is usually secondary to stomach pathology.

- Current symptoms: admit immediately.
- If the symptoms have settled: arrange urgent endoscopy.
- Stop NSAIDs.

OCCULT BLEEDING

This is suggested by anaemia with positive faecal occult bloods.

- Refer routinely.
- Stop NSAIDs.
- Treat with oral iron if iron deficiency anaemia is confirmed.

DIVERTICULITIS

Diverticulitis usually presents with: • lower abdominal pain (usually left iliac fossa) • altered bowel habit • fever.

There may also be • nausea and vomiting • dysuria and urgency (if the affected area lies close to the bladder) • rectal bleeding.

Management

- Mild symptoms: prescribe co-amoxiclav or metronidazole and ciprofloxacin for 7–10 days. Symptoms should improve within 2–3 days.
- Admit if there is: • high fever • significant peritoneal signs • inability to tolerate fluids.
- Exclude, if appropriate, other causes of rectal bleeding, abdominal pain or altered bowel habit, particularly carcinoma of the larger bowel.

INFLAMMATORY BOWEL DISEASE

Diagnosis, treatment and management of exacerbations fall to the specialist. The GP's role is in the management of established disease only.

The inflammation of Crohn's disease affects any part of the GI tract, frequently in discontinuity (skip lesions). Ulcerative colitis is a chronic disease of the colon which always affects the rectum and extends proximally. Drug therapies include oral prednisolone, rectal corticosteroids, aminosalicylates, azathioprine and methotrexate. Antibiotics may be used in Crohn's disease for small intestinal overgrowth, perianal sepsis and abscesses associated with fistulae. Patients with Crohn's disease are more likely to require surgery at some stage.

IRRITABLE BOWEL SYNDROME

Irritable bowel syndrome (IBS) is a functional disorder, which may involve any part of the GI tract. It is characterised by abdominal pain (colonic or dyspeptic) and disordered bowel habit (diarrhoea and constipation occurring alone or in combination). The patient is likely to be young and female, and there is often a variety of non-bowel complaints, e.g. general malaise, headache and backache. Many patients associate an exacerbation of symptoms with stress.

Diagnosis

History

Common symptoms in irritable bowel syndrome

The diagnosis is usually based on history alone. Five symptoms cluster together significantly more frequently than others:

- distension
- relief of pain by defaecation
- looser stools with the onset of pain
- the passage of mucus
- the sensation of incomplete evacuation.

Examination This is normal other than occasional colonic tenderness.

Investigations Hb, ESR and FOBs should all be normal.

Management

Advice
- Improvement with appropriate treatment helps to confirm the diagnosis.
- Discuss the nature of the illness and its relation to stress (relaxation techniques, psychotherapy, etc.).
- Discuss diet:
  - avoid foods which may exacerbate the symptoms (this varies between individuals)
  - encourage a high-fibre diet (see p. 119) and plenty of fluids
  - consider referral to a dietician for e.g. an exclusion diet.

Prescribing
- For constipation: laxitives, e.g. ispaghula husk one sachet in water b.d. after meals.
- For pain:
  - antispasmodics, e.g. mebeverine 135 mg t.d.s. 20 minutes before meals, or peppermint oil 1–2 capsules t.d.s. before meals
  - anticholinergic agents, e.g. amitriptyline 25–75 mg nocte.
- For dysmotility symptoms (e.g. bloating, nausea): metoclopramide 10 mg t.d.s. p.r.n. or domperidone 10–20 mg 4–8-hourly.
- For diarrhoea: e.g. codeine phosphate 30 mg 3–4 times daily.

> **Referral in irritable bowel syndrome**
> Patients should be referred if:
>
> - they are aged >40, with recent onset of symptoms
> - there are other significant symptoms, e.g. weight loss, blood loss, nocturnal symptoms
> - the diagnosis is in doubt.

COELIAC DISEASE

The prevalence of coeliac disease in adults is one in 300. Diagnosis requires a high index of suspicion. It is often wrongly diagnosed as irritable bowel syndrome. In children it commonly presents as growth retardation or delayed puberty. In adults the common presentations are anaemia, chronic fatigue and variable abdominal symptoms (discomfort, bloating, excess wind and an altered bowel habit). It should be considered especially if the patient also has: a family history of coeliac disease, diabetes, an autoimmune disease, osteoporosis, infertility or an undefined neurological disorder. Coeliac disease doubles the risk of GI tumours.

Diagnosis

Investigations

- Take blood for endomysial antibodies (positive predictive value ≥95%) and IgA antibodies (patients with IgA deficiency have a false-negative endomysial antibody result). Antigliadin antibodies are also useful. Refer to a gastroenterologist if results are positive.
- The definitive test is a distal duodenal biopsy.

Bone density scans are recommended at diagnosis, at the menopause for women, at age 55 for men, or if a fragility fracture occurs at any age (coeliac disease increases the risk of osteoporosis).

Management

A strict life-long gluten-free diet.

Prescription charge exemption Patients receiving gluten-free products on prescription are exempt from prescription charges.

CONSTIPATION

Constipation is the passage of hard stools less frequently than the patient's own normal pattern. Ensure that the patient has no misconceptions about normal bowel habits and that the constipation requires treatment. Laxatives should generally be avoided, but if they are used, prolonged treatment is seldom necessary.

In children, a high-fibre/high-fluid diet is often sufficient treatment (see p. 84).

CHRONIC CONSTIPATION

Diagnosis

History A good history is not always easy to obtain, as faecal build up is often very gradual.

Examination Perform an abdominal and rectal examination.

Management

Advice
- Encourage exercise.
- Encourage a high fluid intake.
- Allow sufficient time for defaecation, e.g. after meals (especially after breakfast, when colonic activity is at its highest).
- Encourage a high-fibre diet, e.g. fruit, vegetables, wholemeal bread, pasta, wheat bran, cereals, pulses.

Prescribing
- Stimulants, e.g. senna 2–8 tablets nocte, according to response, are useful for 'getting things going' on an intermittent basis.
- Bulk-forming agents, e.g. ispaghula husk, are rarely necessary if the diet is high in fibre. They are useful for patients with colostomies, ileostomies, haemorrhoids, anal fissure, IBS, etc.
- Osmotic agents, e.g. lactulose 15 ml b.d. retain fluid in the bowel, and are commonly used.
- Stool softeners, e.g. liquid paraffin and magnesium hydroxide emulsion 20 ml p.r.n., may be used.

Referral Refer for exclusion of a more serious underlying pathology if the history suggests it, e.g. constipation developing suddenly in a middle-aged person for no clear reason (see p. 114).

ACUTE CONSTIPATION

The basic advice remains the same as above.

- Try to anticipate the problem, e.g. postoperative, bed-bound, perianal pain, opiates.
- Use senna in sufficient dosage: 6–8 tablets nocte.

- Patients may require disimpaction, especially if they are in pain:
  - insert a glycerol or a sodium phosphate suppository, *or*
  - arrange (usually via the district nurse) for an enema or manual evacuation.
- Enemas:
  - mild: arachis oil enema (to soften impacted faeces) or sodium citrate microenema
  - more powerful: sodium phosphate enema.

JAUNDICE

The common causes of jaundice in adults are: viral hepatitis (see p. 190), alcoholic hepatitis and biliary obstruction due to gallstones or malignancy.

Investigations
- Test the urine for urobilinogen (which indicates haemolysis) and for bilirubin (found in hepatitis and obstruction).
- Take blood for LFTs, hepatitis A, B and C serology, FBC and coagulation screen.
- If obstruction is a possibility, arrange an ultrasound of the liver, gallbladder and pancreas. If obstruction is confirmed, refer.

DERMATOLOGY

BENIGN SUPERFICIAL LUMPS

Benign superficial lesions, including moles, seborrhoeic warts, skin tags and sebaceous cysts, can be removed easily in the surgery by one or other of the following: curettage, cautery, cryotherapy or excision.

SKIN MALIGNANCIES

MALIGNANT MELANOMA

A GP might expect to see one malignant melanoma every 5 years in a list size of 2000 patients. The only effective treatment for melanoma is excision. It is therefore essential that an early diagnosis is made, while the tumour is still thin. Melanomas are extremely fast growing, developing over only a few months.

Diagnosis

History Ask about the following risk factors:
- A mole changing in shape or colour.
- Large numbers of normal naevi, particularly with a family history of malignant melanoma.
- A past history of primary malignant melanoma or severe sunburn.
- General skin type: people with blonde/red hair colour and poorly tanning skin are at greater risk.

Examination

Major features strongly suggestive of malignancy

- Change in size or new lesion.
- Irregular shape.
- Irregular colour.

Also look for other suspicious features, e.g.: • inflammation • crusting or bleeding • changes in sensation.

Management

All suspicious moles should be referred immediately for excision.

Patients with clearly benign lesions should be reassured, and prevention should be discussed; excise the lesion if appropriate.

Long-term prevention High-risk patients should be advised to examine themselves regularly and to know the signs of malignancy. They should protect themselves from the sun, avoid sunbeds and use sunscreens that protect against UVA and UVB with a sun protection factor of >15, e.g. Uvistat 20. Sunscreens can be prescribed on FP10 only for patients with photodermatoses who require high protection (SPF > 15). Prescriptions should be marked with 'ACBS' (Advisory Committee on Borderline Substances).

Low-risk patients should also be advised to protect themselves from the sun and to use sunscreens with an SPF of at least 10.

SOLAR KERATOSES

These are more common on sun-damaged skin and in the elderly. They look like dry, cracked plaques. They have very low malignant potential, and can be treated with cryotherapy or 5-fluorouracil cream b.d. for 1–2 weeks.

BASAL CELL CARCINOMA (RODENT ULCER) AND SQUAMOUS CELL CARCINOMA

These are commonly related to sun exposure. They both have raised irregular edges and may be ulcerated. The BCC may have a pearly border. These should be referred early for excision, radiotherapy or cryotherapy.

ACNE

More then half of British teenagers develop acne severe enough to warrant therapy. Acne can cause great emotional distress, and is usually easily treatable. Sensitivity and understanding are important. Most sufferers will have already self-treated with OTC preparations.

Diagnosis

History Ask about past and present OTC and prescribed treatments.

Examination Look for comedones, erythematous papules and pustules on the face, chest or back. There may be pitted scars.

Management

Most patients need to be reassured that their acne is very largely unrelated to the nature of their diet.

Mild acne These topical preparations should be applied twice daily to clean skin and are likely to cause some degree of skin irritation initially.

- Benzoyl peroxide (1–10%) is useful in inflammatory and non-inflammatory acne. Start treatment with lower strength preparations.
- Topical retinoids (e.g. tretinoin): if, after 4 weeks, response to benzoyl peroxide is insufficient, topical retinoids may be used in addition. If used together, apply each once a day at different times. These are effective against non-inflamed lesions (comedones).
- Topical antibiotics (clindamycin, erythromycin or tetracycline): these are useful in inflammatory acne.
- Azelaic acid is useful in inflammatory and non-inflammatory acne.

Moderate acne

Oral antibiotics These may be used in addition to topical treatments. Improvement may take up to 6 weeks and maximum improvement occurs at 3–4 months. It is worth trying an alternative oral antibiotic if the response to the first is inadequate after 2–3 months. Treatment may continue for several years, if necessary.

- Oxytetracycline 500 mg b.d. for 3 months, then reduced to 250 mg b.d.
- Erythromycin 500 mg b.d. for 3 months, then reduced to 250 mg b.d. (Both antibiotics can be increased to 1–2 g per day, if necessary.)
- Minocycline and doxycycline are significantly more expensive. They are less affected by food.

The combined oral contraceptive in acne

The COC can be started in a patient who has been taking long-term antibiotics for acne without the need for extra contraceptive precautions. If the patient is already on the COC when first starting antibiotics for acne, or when switching to a different antibiotic, additional contraception should be used for the first 2 weeks to allow antibiotic resistance to develop among the bowel flora which are responsible for recycling oestrogens.

Hormonal treatment
- Dianette: this contains cyproterone acetate, an antiandrogen. It is also effective as an oral contraceptive and, if used as such, a prescription charge can be avoided by writing 'for contraception' on the prescription.
- COC: acne may improve with the use of oestrogen-dominant COCs, e.g. Marvelon, and may be exacerbated by the use of predominantly progestogenic preparations.

Severe acne (Also acne that fails to respond to the above treatment.) Refer for oral isotretinoin. This is expensive, teratogenic and has a high side-effect profile.

HIDRADENITIS SUPPURATIVA

This causes chronic papules and pustules, with scarring, in the axillae and/or groins. It can be treated with long-term oxytetracycline 500 mg b.d. Some patients require plastic surgery.

ROSACEA

This is characterised by chronic, shiny facial erythema, especially over the cheeks and central forehead. There may be papules and pustules. It occurs most commonly in middle-aged women. It can be treated with long-term oxytetracycline 250 mg b.d., reducing, if possible, to a maintenance dose of 250 mg daily. Metronidazole gel applied twice daily is an alternative treatment.

 Topical steroids aggravate rosacea.

BACTERIAL SKIN INFECTIONS

CELLULITIS/ERYSIPELAS (STREPTOCOCCAL)

These two conditions may co-exist. Erysipelas is a superficial infection, causing sharply demarcated tender erythematous areas. Cellulitis causes deeper infection, involving the subcutaneous tissues. Treatment is with oral or intramuscular penicillin or erythromycin. Advise bed rest. Occasionally, admission may be required for treatment with intravenous antibiotics.

BOILS (STAPHYLOCOCCAL)

See page 189.

FOLLICULITIS (STAPHYLOCOCCAL)

This is sometimes seen in patients treated with topical steroid ointments for eczema, and as a result of shaving. It should be treated with mild antiseptics, e.g. povidone-iodine, or, if severe, with oral flucloxacillin.

IMPETIGO

Impetigo is a common infectious condition of the skin, caused by *Staphylococcus*.

Diagnosis

History Impetigo starts as a slough, which hardens to form a yellow crust. It is usually painless and occurs anywhere on the body.

It often complicates other skin problems that involve a breach of the skin surface, e.g. cracked lips, cold sores, eczema or grazes.

Examination Look for the yellow crusty lesions sometimes on a weeping, erythematous base. The underlying skin condition may be obvious, but cold sores can be indistinguishable from the impetigo.

Management

- Fusidic acid ointment t.d.s. rubbed on the crusts will help to soften them and prevent the further multiplication of bacteria.
- For widespread or stubborn lesions, use flucloxacillin 250 mg q.d.s for 5 days.
- Erythromycin is effective in patients allergic to penicillin.

> Inform the patient that impetigo is contagious and an individual towel and flannel should be used. It is not necessary to avoid school once treatment has started.

ERYTHRASMA

This usually presents as a brown, slightly scaly area in the armpits or groins. It is asymptomatic and is produced by a *Corynebacterium*. It can be treated with topical imidazoles, e.g. miconazole, or fusidic acid (Fucidin), or with a 2-week course of oral erythromycin.

VIRAL SKIN INFECTIONS

WARTS

Diagnosis

Look for firm papules with a rough hyperkeratotic surface. Plantar warts (verrucae) may look like callosities (hyperkeratosis) and often have a dark centre. They can cause pain on walking.

Management

> Warts and verrucae usually resolve spontaneously, the patient's immune response overcoming the infection. Treatment is only necessary if the patient is troubled by the wart.

Treat with the daily application of a wart paint or gel containing e.g. salicylic acid (e.g. Salactol), having softened the wart in hot water for a few minutes and removed any dead tissue with an emery board or pumice stone. The paint should not touch surrounding healthy tissue. The treatment may need to be continued for 3 months.

Cryotherapy with liquid nitrogen can be used for warts resistant to wart paints. It is quite painful and therefore best avoided in small children. Warn the patient that a blister may occur after treatment. Multiple warts normally require more than one application, and the optimum interval between treatments is 3–4 weeks. Occasionally, resistant warts require treatment with curettage and cautery.

Planar warts should be left to resolve spontaneously, as they are difficult to treat effectively.

Children with verrucae should be allowed to use swimming pools, particularly if the verruca is covered with a plaster, or a water-resistant gel (e.g. Salatac), or if a verruca sock (available OTC) is used.

For genital warts, see page 47.

MOLLUSCUM CONTAGIOSUM

This consists of asymptomatic crops of firm, pink, pearly papules, some of which have a central depression. They resolve spontaneously usually after about 9 months, but occasionally they persist for up to 5 years. Resolution may be hastened by:

- Squeezing each lesion in order to expel the central plug. (Parents of young children with molluscum can be advised to perform this.)
- Cryotherapy.
- Pricking the centre of each lesion with phenol on the end of a cocktail stick.

FUNGAL SKIN INFECTIONS

RINGWORM (TINEA)

This can involve feet (athlete's foot), body, groin, scalp and nails. It is usually indirectly acquired as a result of contact with fungal hyphae in keratin debris. Athlete's foot is frequently the source of groin ringworm.

Diagnosis

Examination

- *Tinea pedis* usually starts with macerated, irritable skin between the toes and may spread to the soles and dorsum of the foot.
- *Tinea corporis* is characterised by red, circular, slightly scaly lesions which clear centrally and spread from the perimeter.
- *Tinea cruris* presents as a well-demarcated, red, slightly scaly groin rash, and is most common in young men.
- *Tinea unguium* causes thickened, yellow friable nails, and most commonly affects one or a few nails only.

Investigation Send off skin scrapings, sub-ungual scrapings or plucked hair, as appropriate, for microscopy. (Unfortunately, results are often negative despite the presence of *Tinea*.)

Management

Skin Keep the affected skin clean and dry. Treat with a topical imidazole cream, e.g. clotrimazole, econazole or miconazole (apply 2–3 times daily, continuing for 14 days after the lesions have healed). Resistant cases can be treated with e.g. oral terbinafine 250 mg daily for 2–6 weeks or itraconazole 200 mg b.d. for 7 days.

Nails Most treatments need to be continued until the affected nails grow out (6 months for fingernails and 12–18 months for toenails).

Topical treatments
- Tioconazole nail solution: apply twice daily.
- Amorolfine nail lacquer: apply 1–2 times weekly.

Oral treatments
- Terbinafine 250 mg daily is expensive, but only needs to be continued for 6 weeks for fingernails and 3 months for toenails.
- 'Pulsed' treatment can be prescribed, e.g. itraconazole 200 mg b.d. for 7 days and subsequent courses repeated after 21-day interval; fingernails two courses, toenails three courses.

CANDIDA INFECTION

Buccal mucosa This is common in babies. Treatment is with e.g. nystatin oral suspension 100 000 units q.d.s. after food or amphotericin lozenges 1 q.d.s., both to be continued for 2 days after lesions have resolved.

Nappy rash See page 87.

Intertrigo/angular stomatitis/chronic paronychia Keep the hands dry and use a topical imidazole cream.

PITYRIASIS VERSICOLOR

This is characterised by an area of scaly, confluent macules which are usually asymptomatic and on the trunk, upper arms or legs. Affected patches remain

 Seborrhoeic dermatitis is often confused with eczema.

pale on tanned skin. Use a topical selenium sulphide, e.g. Selsun shampoo, on all affected areas. Leave on the skin for 10 minutes before washing off. Repeat every other night for 3 weeks. Persistence of hypopigmented areas does not signify treatment failure. Alternatively, use an imidazole cream each night for 2–4 weeks. Oral itraconazole 200 mg daily for 7 days is effective.

SEBORRHOEIC DERMATITIS

This usually presents as red, scaly patches in the eyebrows or nasolabial folds. It is commonly associated with a scaly scalp (dandruff) and blepharitis. Use ketoconazole cream b.d. ('SLS' [Selected List Scheme] must be written on the prescription), continuing for a few days after the lesions have healed, and ketoconazole shampoo twice weekly for 2–4 weeks.

PITYRIASIS ROSEA

This is an eruption of pink macules, mainly over the trunk, which are usually distributed in lines parallel to the ribs. No action is required, but a mild topical steroid will relieve irritation. The rash resolves spontaneously in 6–8 weeks.

GENERALISED PRURITUS

Where there is no obvious skin disease, all patients with persistent generalised pruritus should be investigated to exclude an underlying systemic disorder. Scabies is a common cause – burrows can be difficult to see (see p. 134).

Arrange FBC, ESR, LFTs, serum creatine, blood sugar, serum iron, serum thyroxine, urine protein and a chest X-ray.

If no underlying cause is found:

- Use an emollient regularly (see p. 131).
- Consider use of a topical steroid cream and/or an oral antihistamine.

HAIR LOSS

Acute stress is often the trigger for diffuse hair loss. Thyroid disease, iron deficiency and drug side-effects should be excluded. There is no specific treatment other than treating any identifiable underlying cause.

Alopecia areata normally resolves within a few weeks, although episodes may recur.

Androgenic alopecia may be arrested by the use of topical minoxidil, which is only available on private prescription or OTC.

EXCESSIVE SWEATING

GENERALISED

A cause is rarely identified, but consider menopausal flushing, hyperthyroidism or hyperpituitarism, and autonomic neuropathy.

LOCALISED TO THE AXILLAE, PALMS AND SOLES

- Apply 20% aluminium chloride hexahydrate roll-on antiperspirant to dry axillae each night, and reduce to 1–2 times weekly as improvement occurs.
- Smelly feet are usually due to bacterial superinfection of sweat. Treat with e.g. potassium permanganate soaks (1:10 000 aqueous solution) twice daily, until the smell has improved. (Potassium permanganate stains the skin.)
- Axillary odour can be treated with an antiseptic cream, e.g. chlorhexidine cream b.d.
- Consider dermatological referral for iontophoresis, which may help palmar or plantar hyperhydrosis. In intractable cases consider referral for thoracoscopic sympathectomy (also treats severe facial blushing).

ECZEMA

'Eczema' is synonymous with 'dermatitis'. Treatment is basically the same, whether the eczema is exogenous (allergic and contact dermatitis) or endogenous (atopic).

Atopic eczema is not present at birth, but often appears within the first 2 years of life. It usually resolves in childhood, but it may continue into adult life.

Diagnosis
The main symptom is itching. The main signs are redness, papules, vesicles and hyperkeratosis, and there may be weeping and crusting.

Unlike fungal rashes, which have a well-demarcated edge, eczema is more diffuse.

Management

General Sympathetic explanation is essential, especially to the parents of young children with atopic eczema. Assess possible irritants or trigger factors with a view to avoidance, if possible, e.g. contact with metals, detergent or woollen clothing, dietary factors, emotion, heat, cold. If appropriate, give details of local and national support groups (see p. 384). The skin should be kept clean and warm, and prolonged contact with water, detergent, etc., should be avoided. If the hands are affected, gloves should be worn at the sink etc.

Emollients Emollients moisten dry, scaly skin, and are the mainstay of treatment. They can be used at any time on dry skin, but are particularly useful at bathtime, when different preparations can be used in combination: • soap substitute, e.g. emulsifying ointment • bath oil, e.g. Oilatum emollient • emollient cream after bathing, e.g. aqueous cream.

Ointments are more effective than creams, but in view of their greasiness they are less user-friendly.

Topical steroids Aim to use the weakest preparation sufficient to control the disease. Acute exacerbations should be treated with relatively potent steroids. The potency should be quickly reduced when control is gained. Try to avoid anything stronger than 1% hydrocortisone on the face or in infancy.

Steroid potency
- Mildly potent: e.g. hydrocortisone 0.5%, 1% (can be bought OTC for use on all parts of the body except the face) and 2.5%.
- Moderately potent: e.g. clobetasone butyrate 0.05% (Eumovate).
- Potent: e.g. betamethasone 0.1% (Betnovate).
- Very potent: e.g. clobetasol propionate 0.05% (Dermovate).

Other treatments Secondary infection should be treated with topical antibiotic cream or ointment (e.g. fusidic acid) or oral antistaphylococcal antibiotics (e.g. flucloxacillin or erythromycin).

Severe eczema on the limbs can be treated with bandages (wet wrapping) which may be applied overnight on top of steroid ointment or emollients, e.g. zinc paste and icthammol bandage, zinc paste and coal tar bandage or simple elasticated tubular bandage. A community paediatric/eczema nurse may be available to instruct parents on their use.

A sedative antihistamine at night may help itching in exacerbations, e.g. trimeprazine 2 mg /kg for children over 2 years old.

The role of diet in atopic eczema is contentious. Cow's milk is the most commonly implicated food, and should be avoided for the first 6 months of life by children at risk of atopic eczema. Exclusion diets help a small number of children, and should only be undertaken with expert advice from a dietician.

Gamolenic acid in evening primrose oil (Epogam) can be very helpful. However, it is expensive and any benefit is usually small.

PSORIASIS

In total, 1.5% of the population are affected by this chronic inflammatory skin disease during their lifetime. It most commonly presents as multiple, large, well-demarcated, red plaques with thick silvery scales. There is no cure and it is usually life-long, with exacerbations and remissions. The patient should therefore be given detailed information on self-management. The Psoriasis Association can be helpful (see p. 387).

Psoriasis is often exacerbated by trauma, stress or infections.

STABLE PLAQUES

Management

Emollients (see p. 131). These help to control the scaling and irritation, and their use should be encouraged in addition to other treatments.

Salicylic acid This acts as a keratolytic, and is often used in mixtures with tar.

Coal tar This is anti-inflammatory and keratolytic and should be applied twice daily or at night to plaques. Thick pastes and ointments are more effective, but their use is limited by their unpleasant appearance and smell. Thinner creams, e.g. Alphosyl, are more acceptable. Coal tar emollient bath oils, are useful.

Dithranol This is the most potent topical antiplaque preparation, but is difficult to use, as it can cause quite severe skin irritation and staining to skin (if left on for more than 30 minutes), bath and clothes. Preparations such as Dithrocream cause fewer side-effects and are easier to use than the ointments and pastes. Preparations should be applied daily to plaques and washed off after 30 minutes. Old clothes should be worn during application. Start with a low concentration (0.1%) and gradually build up to the maximum concentration which produces a therapeutic effect without irritation (up to 3%).

Calcipotriol (Dovonex) This is a vitamin D derivative and is widely used. It should be applied to plaques twice daily. It does not stain clothing, and does not have an unpleasant smell.

Topical steroids These can be used in stable disease when plaques are few in number. Use a moderately potent or potent steroid. There is a risk of rebound exacerbation and skin thinning if used excessively.

PUVA, oral retinoids, methotrexate, cyclosporin, etc. If psoriasis is extensive or unresponsive to the above treatments, refer for these.

SCALP PSORIASIS

In contrast to the scalp changes of seborrhoeic dermatitis, the scalp lesions in psoriasis are easily felt.

Daily shampooing with coal tar shampoo, e.g. Polytar, is helpful, but by itself is unlikely to control thick plaques. Calcipotriol scalp solution used twice daily, or topical steroid lotions (e.g. Betnovate scalp application) used on a daily basis, or less frequently, may be prescribed in addition.

Mixtures of tar and salicylic acid, although messy, are particularly effective for severe scaling, e.g. Cocois scalp ointment, which should be applied to the scalp once weekly, or more often if necessary, and shampooed off after 1 hour. Mixtures of steroid and salicylic acid, e.g. Diprosalic scalp application, are also helpful.

GUTTATE PSORIASIS

These plaques are round, unlike the oval lesions of pityriasis rosea. They usually clear completely in a few months, but classical psoriasis may develop subsequently.

Perform a throat swab, as guttate psoriasis usually follows a streptococcal throat infection.

Use a mild tar-based cream, e.g. Alphosyl or Alphosyl HC, and consider referral for UVB phototherapy.

KERATOSIS PILARIS

This is a very common disorder where the hair follicles are plugged with keratin, causing rough skin. The commonest sites are the posterior upper arm and the lateral cheeks, and it usually presents in young women as a cosmetic nuisance.

Treat with mild keratolytics, e.g. salicylic acid 2–4% in soft white paraffin, or advise cosmetic exfoliation. Emollients are helpful.

HEAD LICE

Head lice are common, and a particular problem in young schoolchildren and their families. They present as an itchy scalp.

Management

Nit combs

Daily use of nit combs, ideally on wet, conditioned hair, is now advocated in preference to insecticides (particularly if the lice are few in number, or have shown resistance to insecticides), in order to eliminate new lice and therefore to break the cycle. Nit combs can remove lice at all stages of development. They will not remove empty egg-cases, which persist on the hair for some time.

Insecticides clear the lice at all stages except the very young eggs. The treatments should therefore be repeated after an interval of 7–10 days.

Lotions should be used in preference to shampoos, which are relatively ineffective. Use e.g. permethrin cream rinse. Rub into damp hair and rinse after 10 minutes.

Resistance to insecticides is becoming increasingly common. If a course of treatment fails to cure, a different insecticide should be used for the next course. Insecticides can be bought OTC. Essential oils, e.g. tea tree oil, may be used, mixed with shampoo prior to nit-combing, to help clearance. All members of a household should be treated. Parents should notify the school so that all members of the class can be treated.

SCABIES

Scabies spreads by skin to skin contact, e.g. holding hands with an infected person or sleeping in the same bed. It can take up to 6 weeks to develop symptoms after being infected. All household members and intimate contacts should be treated, to avoid reinfection. Commonly there are just a few mites on the skin, creating burrows, but the allergy to them can cause generalised itch and rash.

- Treat with malathion lotion or permethrin cream (available OTC).
- Apply over the whole body from the neck down. Wash off after the recommended time (8–24 hours). Reapply treatment to hands every time they are washed within the treatment period. Reapply the same treatment 7 days after the first application.

- The itch takes 2–3 weeks after treatment to subside. (This can be treated with e.g. crotamitron cream ± hydrocortisone cream.)
- It is not necessary to wash clothes, towels or bedding.

OTHER SKIN INFESTATIONS

BODY LICE

These are uncommon in developed countries and are associated with neglect. They cause generalised pruritus associated with excoriations, and live in clothing, only visiting the skin to feed. Treatment is by washing the clothes in hot water.

CRAB LICE

These are capable of living in all hair except scalp hair, which is too dense for them. The most common site is pubic hair. They are transmitted by close physical contact, usually sexual. Infection of children is not evidence of sexual abuse. Use aqueous preparations of e.g. malathion over the whole body. Instructions for use are as for head lice.

FLEA BITES

These usually present as multiple lesions around the ankles and calves. Often, only one member of the family is affected.

Use hydrocortisone ointment or calamine lotion on spots to relieve the itching (both can be bought OTC). Deflea pets, and spray insecticide on soft furnishings and carpets. Professional exterminators, via the Environmental Health Department, are sometimes needed.

BED BUGS

These are suggested by very large lesions on the face or hands, particularly when new lesions are found each morning. Bed bugs live behind wallpaper and skirting boards, not in beds. The Environmental Health Department should be called to treat the house.

ANIMAL MITES

These are suggested by itchy papules, principally on the abdomen, thighs and arms (i.e. the main sites of contact with an animal sitting on the sufferer's lap). Treat the animal.

ALLERGIC RASHES

It is often difficult to establish a cause; any potential cause should, if possible, be avoided. It *is* possible to become hypersensitive to an allergen after many years of uneventful exposure to it.

Use an oral antihistamine, e.g. loratadine 10 mg o.d. A mild topical steroid helps to relieve pruritus.

CHAPTER 10

CARDIOLOGY

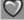

PRIMARY PREVENTION OF CORONARY HEART DISEASE

Primary prevention relates to individuals who have not developed symptomatic coronary heart disease (CHD) or other major atherosclerotic disease.

In order to calculate a patient's CHD risk the following information is required:

- gender
- age
- smoking status
- presence of diabetes
- total cholesterol
- HDL cholesterol
- systolic blood pressure.

Apply this information to the graphs on pages 139–142 to calculate the 10-year risk of developing CHD.

> Patients with a 10-year CHD risk >15% should take aspirin 75 mg o.d. unless contraindicated. Patients with a 10-year CHD risk >30% should, in addition, be prescribed a statin.

General lifestyle advice for prevention of CHD
- Stop smoking (see p. 313).
- Dietary advice:
  - aim for ideal weight (see obesity, p. 104)
  - reduce dietary fats (see cholesterol, p. 145)
  - consume five portions of fruit or vegetables per day.
- Encourage exercise: recommend at least 20 minutes of brisk exercise three times per week.
- Encourage stress reduction (see anxiety, p. 296).
- Avoid excessive alcohol intake (>14 units per week for women and >21 units for men).

Risk factors for CHD
- Male.
- Age >50 years.
- South Asian/Afro-Caribbean race.
- Smoking.
- Obesity.
- Hypertension.
- Diabetes.
- Hyperlipidaemia.

- Other atheromatous disease (CVA/TIA, peripheral vascular disease).
- Family history of premature atheromatous disease.

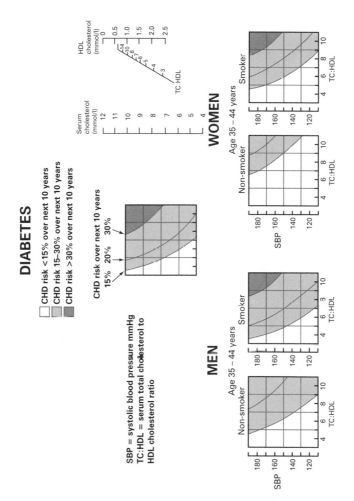

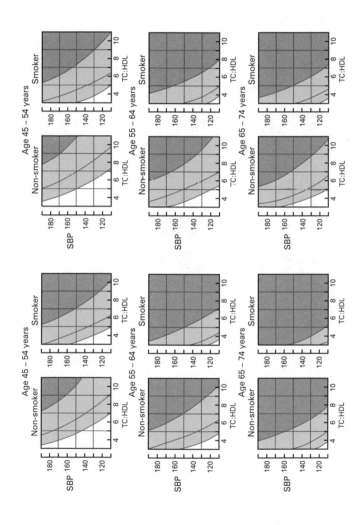

NO DIABETES

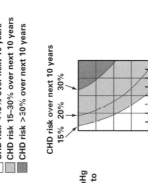

☐ CHD risk <15% over next 10 years
☐ CHD risk 15–30% over next 10 years
☐ CHD risk >30% over next 10 years

CHD risk over next 10 years
15%   20%   30%

SBP = systolic blood pressure mmHg
TC:HDL = serum total cholesterol to
HDL cholesterol ratio

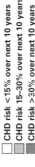

Serum
cholesterol
(mmol/l)

HDL
cholesterol
(mmol/l)

MEN

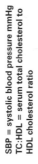

Age 35 – 44 years

Non-smoker

Smoker

WOMEN

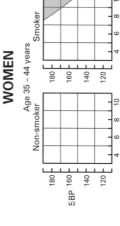

Age 35 – 44 years

Non-smoker

Smoker

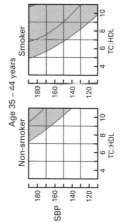

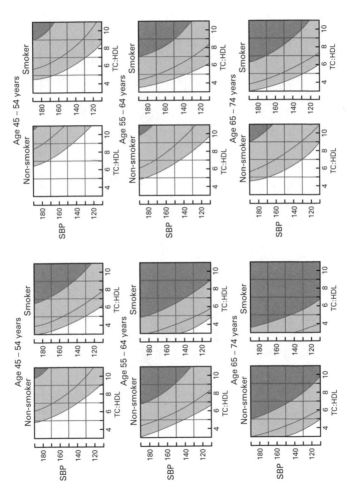

Reproduced from: Joint British recommendations on prevention of coronary heart disease in clinical practice. *Heart* 1998;80(suppl 2):S1–29.

HYPERTENSION

Hypertension affects approximately 15% of the population. It can be managed almost entirely in general practice. The following advice is based on the British Hypertension Society's Guidelines 1999.

Diagnosis

The new hypertensive On finding a raised blood pressure for the first time in a patient, the path described below can be followed.

- <139/89: no treatment, no follow-up (<130/80 in diabetics).
- >160/100: treat if consistently above this level on four or more consecutive readings over 2 weeks.
- Between 140/90 and 160/99: repeat BP reading four times over 3–6 weeks.

> ⚠ **Diastolic BP of >120 and rising on subsequent examinations suggests malignant hypertension. Urgent referral or hospital admission is necessary.**

After the fourth BP reading
- If any diastolic BP is <90 and the systolic is <140, no treatment is indicated (<130/80 in diabetics).
- If the BP is persistently in the range 140–160/90–99:
  - treatment is indicated if the patient is at high risk of cardiovascular disease (>15% 10-year CHD risk, see p. 138), or if there is evidence of target organ damage, as suggested by:
    - left ventricular hypertrophy (CXR or ECG)
    - transient ischaemic attacks
    - previous stroke, angina or MI
    - renal impairment (raised creatinine, proteinuria/haematuria)
    - peripheral vascular disease
    - hypertensive retinopathy.
  - Treatment is not indicated if there is no evidence of target organ disease, and the 10-year CHD risk is <15%. Check the BP (see box on p. 144) and reassess the CHD risk annually.

Initial investigations
- Blood tests: C&E, total cholesterol and HDL cholesterol, urate, fasting plasma glucose.
- Urine tests: protein.
- ECG: for left ventricular hypertrophy.

- Patients under 35 years old: 24-hour urinary metadrenaline for phaeochromocytoma.
- Examine for retinopathy, abdominal aortic aneurysm, renal bruit, absent foot pulses.

Management

Advice All hypertensives should be given advice on non-pharmacological methods.

- See general lifestyle advice (p. 138).

Prescribing
- Drug treatment can be initiated with bendrofluazide 2.5 mg daily.
  – The contraindication to thiazides is gout.
- If thiazides are contraindicated, use atenolol 50 mg daily.
  – The contraindications to beta blockers are: heart failure, asthma, peripheral vascular disease.
- If both the above are contraindicated, use either a calcium-channel blocker,

---

Blood pressure measurement
Use the British Hypertension Society recommendations.

- Use a device that has validated accuracy and that is calibrated and maintained.
- The patient should be seated, with their arm at the level of the heart. The bladder size of the cuff should be appropriate for the size of the arm.
- In older or diabetic patients, standing blood pressure (BP) should also be measured.
- Remove tight clothing, support the arm at heart level and ensure that the hand is relaxed. Apply the appropriate sized cuff.
- The patient should be encouraged to uncross their legs and not to talk whilst the reading is being taken.
- Deflate the cuff slowly at 2 mm per second.
- Read the BP to the nearest 2 mm.
- Measure the diastolic pressure as the disappearance of sounds (phase 5).
- Take two measurements at each visit.
- Use the average for several visits when calculating cardiovascular risk in mild hypertension.
- Many practices will now use electronic sphygmomanometers, but the principles remain the same.
- Ambulatory BP monitoring may be indicated to diagnose 'white coat hypertension', excessive variability, suspected hypotension and resistance to drug therapy.

such as amlodipine 5 mg o.d. or an ACE inhibitor, such as lisinopril 2.5 mg o.d. initially.
- Start aspirin 75 mg o.d. in patients over 50 years old with satisfactory blood pressure control, if there is target organ damage or diabetes or established cardiovascular disease or if the 10-year CHD risk is greater than 15%.
- Start statin (e.g. Simvastatin) in patients under 75 years old when serum total cholesterol is >5.0 mmol/l and the 10-year coronary risk is >30%, or if there is established CHD.

Follow-up
- Frequency of follow-up should be 4-weekly initially, unless there is a need to achieve more urgent control (e.g. BP > 200/120).

 If there are unacceptable side-effects, change to an alternative drug.

- Aim for BP of <140/85 ideally, but <150/90 is acceptable (<130/80 in diabetes).
- If control is not achieved, add a second drug. If BP is still above target, increase the dose of the second drug.
- If control is still not achieved, either add a third drug or consider referral (see below).
- Once control is achieved, follow up with BP check every 6 months. Arrange annual urinalysis for protein, and check C&E and fasting blood sugar. Recalculate CHD risk every year.

Reasons for referral
- Malignant hypertension.
- Secondary hypertension (raised creatinine or proteinuria).
- Refractory hypertension (difficult to treat with two or more drugs).
- Hypertension of sudden onset.
- Hypertension that is worsening despite treatment.
- Hypertension under age 35 years with multiple cardiovascular risk factors.
- Pregnancy.

Stopping antihypertensives If BP is consistently <140/85 and there is no evidence of target organ disease, antihypertensives can be gradually withdrawn.
  Regular monitoring is essential and should be long-term.

CHOLESTEROL

High cholesterol is principally a risk factor for the development of cardiovascular disease. GPs should consider the level of a patient's cholesterol when monitoring overall coronary risk.

Diagnosis

Test serum cholesterol if:

- The patient is at high risk of CHD:
  - hypertensive
  - diabetic
  - established atheromatous disease (angina, MI, CABG, CVA, TIA, peripheral vascular disease)
  - combination of risk factors, including smoking, obesity, lack of exercise
  - family history of heart disease: first-degree relative suffering coronary death under age 50 for male relative, age 60 for female relative.
- Family history of hyperlipidaemia.
- Patient's request.

Interpreting results
- Measurements of both total cholesterol and HDL cholesterol should be made (see pp. 139–142).
- Readings should be applied to the Joint British Societies Coronary Risk Prediction Chart to assess 10-year coronary risk (see pp. 139–142).
- Very high serum cholesterol (say, >10) suggests a familial hyperlipidaemia.
- Serum cholesterol is elevated in:
  - diabetes mellitus
  - nephrotic syndrome
  - hypothyroidism
  - pregnancy.

Management

Advice
- Give dietary advice:
  - to achieve ideal weight
  - to reduce overall fat intake
  - to reduce saturated fat intake.
- Give advice on other risk factors (see p. 138).
- In the absence of established cardiovascular disease, treat patients under 75 years old with a statin if the 10-year coronary risk is greater than 30% (see p. 144).

> Patients with a history of MI or angina, CVA/TIA or peripheral vascular disease should be started on a statin (e.g. Simvastatin starting at 20 mg o.n.) to achieve a total cholesterol <5.0 mmol/l or a 20–25% reduction, whichever is the lower value.

> **Dietary measures**
> (Send the patient to the practice nurse for advice.)
>
> - Explain the role of diet in heart disease and the need for change.
> - Measure weight and height and calculate body mass index from the formula BMI = weight (kg)/(height (m))^2. Aim for a BMI of <25 for men and <23 for women.
> - Ask the patient to keep an accurate dietary diary for 1 week.
> - Review the diary with the patient, identifying sources of saturated fat intake.
> - Suggest low-fat alternatives, aiming to substitute polyunsaturated fats or carbohydrates for saturated fats.
> - Encourage compliance. Offer a follow-up appointment.

- Total cholesterol over 10mmol/l: refer to the lipid clinic.

Follow-up
- At 3-monthly intervals, initially.
- If the serum cholesterol level is reduced, reinforce dietary measures and concentrate on other risk factors for cardiovascular disease.
- Check LFTs at the first follow-up if a statin has been started.
- Titrate the dose of statin to achieve target cholesterol.
- Remember the coronary risk rises with age. Reassessment of risk level may indicate treatment at some point in the future. Plan to reassess the patient at a suitable interval.

INTERMITTENT CLAUDICATION

Intermittent claudication is often a sign of more widespread atheromatous disease, which should be sought.

Diagnosis

History Ask about pain in the legs on walking, which is relieved by rest. The calves are usually affected.

Risk factors: • smoking • hypertension • diabetes • established atheromatous disease.

Examination This may be normal, but:
- Look for cold 'feet', no hair on legs, dry or flaky skin.
- Check BP and peripheral pulses.
- Check the feet for corns, fungal infections, badly cut nails.

Investigations As for general atheromatous disease, i.e.: • cholesterol • fasting blood glucose • ECG.

Management
- Document the distance at which claudication begins.
- Involve a podiatrist.
- Consider aspirin and statins (see p. 144).

Advice
- See general lifestyle advice (p. 138).
- Ask patient to report early signs of damage to the feet, e.g. blisters.

Referral If this general advice fails to help, refer to vascular surgical outpatients for consideration for angiography to assess the arterial supply to the legs.

CHEST PAIN

The causes of chest pain can range from minor musculoskeletal aches to life-threatening cardiac ischaemia. Surprisingly, both conditions are relatively common in general practice.

Diagnosis

History In diagnosing chest pain a good history is essential, especially if the initial contact is over the telephone.

The first question to ask yourself is, 'Is it an emergency?', i.e.:

- **myocardial infarction**
- **dissecting aneurysm**
- **pulmonary embolus.**

Ask about:

- The nature of the pain, e.g. central, crushing, tight pain, radiating to arms or neck suggests MI, whereas central, tearing pain radiating to the back suggests dissection. PE causes pleuritic pain and often shortness of breath.
- The patient's appearance: collapsed, pale or grey, breathless and sweaty all suggest serious pathology.
- Risk factors for MI and dissecting aneurysm: see risk factors for CHD (p. 138).
- Risk factors for PE:
  - recent DVT
  - surgery
  - trauma
  - combined pill

– smoking
– history of thrombosis
– long-haul flight (economy-class syndrome).

 If the patient is unwell or the history suggests an MI, immediate admission to hospital is essential.

If the initial impression is of non-urgent pathology, a more leisurely history and examination can be performed.

The main differential diagnosis then includes: ● oesophagitis/reflux ● angina/MI ● costochondral/musculoskeletal pain ● chest infection/tracheitis.

A detailed account of the nature of the patient's pain, including site, character, onset, duration, aggravating and relieving factors, associated symptoms and recent past medical history will usually provide a diagnosis.

Examination
● General appearance.
● Pulse.
● BP.
● Temperature.
● Chest, heart and abdomen. Do not forget to press on the chest wall to elicit musculoskeletal pain (common).
● Listen for the friction rub of pericarditis (rare).
● Epigastric tenderness suggests gastritis/reflux.

Investigations
● ECG: this may show evidence of acute MI or ischaemia, but may also be normal in both these conditions.
● CXR: this is of little diagnostic value, but it may confirm a chest infection, fractured rib or rib metastases.

The diagnosis often remains unclear at this stage. The confusion is usually between myocardial ischaemia and oesophagitis/reflux.

A therapeutic trial of either an antacid/H$_2$ blocker or a nitrate/beta blocker is then justified, e.g.:

● magnesium trisilicate 20 ml p.r.n. or cimetidine 400 mg b.d., or
● GTN sublingual p.r.n. or atenolol 100 mg o.d.

The choice is governed by the 'best guess' based on the history and examination so far.

Follow-up If the diagnosis is still in doubt after 24–48 hours on a therapeutic trial, referral to the cardiology outpatient clinic for the purpose of reaching a diagnosis can be justified. The following pages outline the management of ischaemic chest pain once a diagnosis has been reached.

ANGINA

Angina is pain due to myocardial ischaemia.

Diagnosis

History Ask about:
- The nature of the pain: central, tight or constricting, radiating to the arms or neck?
- Aggravating factors: exertion, walking uphill or into the wind, cold weather, large meals?
- Relieving factors: rest, nitrates?
- Risk factors (see p. 138).

Examination Expect this to be normal. Look for: ● heart failure (ankles, lung bases and JVP) ● arrhythmias/murmurs.

Investigations
- FBC: anaemia may unmask angina.
- ECG: a baseline ECG may be helpful for future reference, but expect this to be normal.
- CXR: this is unhelpful unless heart failure is suspected.

> At this stage the diagnosis should fall into one of four groups:
>
> - uncertain diagnosis (see p. 148)
> - stable angina
> - unstable angina
> - suspected MI (see p. 151).

STABLE ANGINA

This is angina that is predictable, i.e. the symptoms are brought on by similar amounts of exercise every time; they are relieved by rest; and there is no change in the frequency of the attacks.

Management

Advice See general lifestyle advice (p. 138). Warn the patient to report any increase in chest pain immediately.

Prescribing Nitrates are the mainstay of treatment. Start with:

- Sublingual or buccal preparation, e.g. one or two GTN tablets p.r.n. (Warn of headache.)
- Oral nitrates can be prescribed if the patient requires a regular daily dose of the sublingual preparation, e.g. isosorbide mononitrate 10–20 mg t.d.s.
- Beta blockers, e.g. atenolol 50–100 mg o.d., can also be added if there is no evidence of heart failure.

If patients on the above medication require more medical treatment, or if there are contraindications to the above, the calcium-channel blockers are useful, e.g. amlodipine 5–10 mg o.d. or diltiazem 60 m t.d.s.

 All patients with angina should take aspirin 75 mg daily, unless containicated, and a statin.

Referral Refer for exercise ECG/angiography as a routine outpatient referral.

Follow-up Continue lifestyle advice and attention to other risk factors.

UNSTABLE ANGINA

This is angina that has grown worse/more frequent over the previous month or less. Particularly worrying are rest pain and nocturnal pain.

Management

 Discuss with the cardiology team with a view to an urgent outpatient appointment or admission.

Otherwise the management is as for stable angina.

ACUTE MYOCARDIAL INFARCTION (MI)

 Call 999 and request ambulance paramedics as soon as an acute MI is suspected, even if this is before the patient has been seen.

This is a true general practice emergency, for which immediate action has been shown to reduce mortality. Among a GP's 2000 patients there will be two episodes of acute MI per year.

Diagnosis

History Ask about:
- the nature of the pain, e.g. central, crushing, tight chest pain radiating to arms or neck
- associated features, e.g. nausea, breathlessness, sweatiness, palpitations
- risk factors (see p. 138).

Examination The general appearance is usually of an anxious, slightly sweaty patient.

Check the blood pressure and pulse to assess for cardiac output and arrhythmias. Examine for signs of heart failure. The heart sounds are usually unchanged.

Investigations
- ECG: if an ECG machine (or a defibrillator with cardiac monitor) is available, it is worth connecting it up, but this must not delay the calling of the ambulance. If the diagnosis is in doubt, a normal ECG will not rule out an acute MI.
- Cardiographic monitoring is most useful in the acute situation for the detection and treatment of arrhythmias.

If the diagnosis is in doubt, see: chest pain, diagnosis (p. 148).

Immediate management of suspected MI
- Reassure the patient.
- Make sure the ambulance has been called.
- Site an intravenous cannula.
- Give pain relief intravenously, e.g. diamorphine 2.5–5 mg or morphine 5–10 mg (the dose being titrated against the patient's response) with an antiemetic (e.g. prochlorperazine 12.5 mg i.v. or metoclopramide 10 mg i.v.).
- For heart failure give frusemide 40 mg i.v.
- For hypotension (systolic pressure <100 mmHg) with bradycardia (<50) give atropine 300 µg i.v. Repeat at 5-minute intervals to a maximum dose of 1.2 mg.
- Give aspirin 300 mg, unless the patient is allergic to aspirin.
- Await the arrival of the ambulance and be prepared for the risk of cardiac arrest. Check the BP and cardiac rhythm regularly.
- Telephone the hospital to inform the medical team of the patient's imminent arrival. If there is time before the ambulance departs, write a

covering letter, listing the time of onset of symptoms, drugs given and cardiac history.

Late presentation of MI
- If less than 24 hours have elapsed, admit the patient.
- If more than 24 hours have elapsed since the onset of severe chest pain, it is not essential to admit the patient, as long as there are no remaining symptoms or signs.
- If the patient is kept at home, examine regularly for signs of heart failure. Confirm diagnosis by taking bloods for cardiac enzymes. See post-myocardial infarction, below.

Follow-up
See post-myocardial infarction, below.

Administration
Claim for the cost of supplying and personally administering injectables on FP10 (GP10 in Scotland).

POST-MYOCARDIAL INFARCTION

The aim of primary care after an acute MI is to support the patient and family in rehabilitation and secondary prevention.

Diagnosis

Examination Look for:
- arrhythmias, hypotension, murmurs, signs of heart failure
- the psychological effects of MI, which include
  - depression
  - beta blocker side-effects
  - fear of physical exertion
  - insecurity
  - pessimism.

 Pay attention to risk factors (see also p. 138)

Management

Advice The patient should aim to return to normal activities by 6 weeks. This includes driving and sex. Graduated increase in the level of exercise should be limited by pain or tiredness. Regular daily exercise should be encouraged.

Prescribing Ensure that the patient is taking both:

- aspirin 75–150 mg o.d. (unless allergic)
- a beta blocker, e.g. atenolol 50 mg o.d. (unless in heart block)
- a statin
- an ACE inhibitor.

Check the patient understands the importance of long-term compliance.

HEART FAILURE

Congestive cardiac failure is a clinical syndrome of shortness of breath, fatigue and fluid retention. It affects about 1–3% of the population.

> Swelling of the ankles is a common general practice symptom. The commonest cause is dependent oedema due to venous insufficiency. Once heart failure has been excluded, treat with support stockings and elevate the legs. A mild diuretic such as bendrofluazide 2.5 mg o.d. may be used if necessary.

Diagnosis
There are two aspects: diagnosing heart failure and diagnosing its cause.

History Ask about:
- Symptoms of heart failure:
  - shortness of breath
  - orthopnoea
  - paroxysmal nocturnal dyspnoea
  - swollen ankles
  - fatigue.
- Possible causes of heart failure:
  - past MI
  - past heart surgery
  - anaemia
  - thyrotoxicosis
  - arrhythmia
  - CHD
  - NSAIDs (fluid retention)
  - beta blockers (decreased myocardial contractility).

Examination Look for:
- Signs of heart failure:
  - raised jugular venous pulse

    – basal crackles

    – swollen ankles.

- Possible causes of heart failure:
  - irregular pulse: arrhythmia
  - tachycardia, exophthalmos: thyrotoxicosis
  - raised BP: hypertensive disease
  - murmur: valvular heart disease
  - pallor: anaemia.
- Signs of associated cardiovascular disease:
  - carotid bruits
  - absence of peripheral pulses.

Investigations Consider:

- Bloods:
  - FBC: anaemia
  - TFT: thyrotoxicosis
  - U&E: prior to treatment
  - LFT: can be disordered in heart failure.
- CXR:
  - left ventricular hypertrophy/aneurysm
  - cardiomegaly.
- ECG:
  - LVH
  - arrhythmia
  - tachycardia
  - MI.
- Echocardiogram (by referral) for all patients, where resources allow, but especially in the following:
  - patient under 65
  - murmur (may need surgery)
  - severe symptoms
  - uncertain diagnosis or cause
  - acute onset (admit – see above).

Management

Treat the underlying cause specifically, if possible.

Advice See page 138.

Prescribing

To control symptoms Frusemide 20–40 mg mane for moderate symptoms.

To improve prognosis ACE inhibitors, e.g. lisinopril 2.5–20 mg o.d.

Method of starting ACE inhibition
- Check C&E.
- Omit diuretics on the morning of initiating therapy.

Is the patient in acute left ventricular failure? If so, treat as an emergency:

- **Give:**
  - **diamorphine 2.5–5 mg i.v.**
  - **frusemide 40 mg i.v.**
  - **GTN sublingually**
  - **O$_2$ when available.**
- **Sit the patient up to decrease pulmonary oedema.**
- **Consider admission.**

- Increase the dose by a factor of 2 every week, if tolerated. Check C&E at 2 weeks and BP with every dose increase.
- Avoid potassium-sparing diuretics and potassium supplements.

Follow-up
- Regular review, probably 6-monthly, but depends on the severity and underlying cause.
- Continued lifestyle advice and encouragement.
- Consider stopping treatment if the underlying cause is corrected.

RAYNAUD'S PHENOMENON

Raynaud's phenomenon is characterised by cold, blue fingers after exposure to cold. It can be caused by vibration, e.g. driving, and can also affect the toes.

Management
- Reassure the patient it is not dangerous.
- Encourage the patient to stop smoking.
- Advise keeping the hands warm, using gloves if necessary.
- Nifedipine 10 mg t.d.s. can be used if the symptoms are severe. Increase to 20 mg t.d.s. if there is no response after 1 week.
- Surgery: sympathectomy may help severe disease.

 Consider other connective tissue disorders, e.g. scleroderma, systemic sclerosis.

 Treat any underlying disease which may be associated, e.g. peripheral vascular disease (see p. 147).

FUNNY TURNS

Syncope is characterised by transient loss of consciousness, with or without a fall.
Simple vasovagal faints are the commonest cause of syncope in young patients.
The phrase 'funny turn' is often used by patients and relations to describe a wide
variety of symptoms, which include syncope (see dizziness, p. 276).

The causes can be divided as follows.

Non-pathological • Faints • cough/micturition syncope.

Cardiovascular • Arrhythmia • valvular • postural hypotension •
vertebrobasilar insufficiency.

Neurological • TIA/CVA • epilepsy.

Other • Hypoglycaemia.

Diagnosis

History Ask about:
- Preceding symptoms:
    - palpitations (arrhythmia)
    - aura (epilepsy)
    - emotional stress (faint)
    - cough/micturition (syncope)
    - chest pain (ischaemia).
- Witnessed account:
    - ?tonic/clonic
    - ?tongue-biting
    - ?asymmetrical weakness
    - ?urinary incontinence (epilepsy)
    - post-ictal drowsiness.
- Drug history (for postural hypotension): diuretics, nitrates, tricyclics,
  antihypertensives, sedatives, hypnotics, neuroleptics.
- Family history of sudden death: ?cardiomyopathy.

Examination Look for:
- Cardiovascular:
    - pulse (?irregular)
    - BP (?postural drop)
    - heart sounds (?aortic stenosis)
    - carotids (?bruits)
    - extend neck (causes faintness in vertebrobasilar insufficiency).
- Central nervous system:
    - ?post-ictal
    - ?residual CVA/TIA deficit.

Investigations
- FBC.
- C&E (if on digoxin/diuretics).
- Blood glucose.
- ECG.

Management

Treatment The following are treatable in general practice:
- Postural hypotension:
  – advise the patient to rise slowly
  – surgical stockings
  – change responsible drugs if possible.
- Some arrhythmias (see below).
- Vertebrobasilar insufficiency:
  – explain the symptoms
  – advise the patient to avoid sudden neck movements.
- TIAs:
  – aspirin 75–150 mg daily
  – identify cause (e.g. AF).
- Hypoglycaemia:
  – if known diabetic: glucose orally or i.v. (50 ml of 50% solution)
  – may need to adjust daily insulin dose.

Referral
- TIA: for carotid flow studies.
- Some arrhythmias (see below).
- Valvular heart disease.
- New or poorly controlled epilepsy.
- Unexplained loss of consciousness. (Refer either to a cardiologist or neurologist.)

Recurrent syncope
- Is the diagnosis correct?
- Advise the patient to avoid dangerous situations.
- The patient should inform the Driver and Vehicle Licensing Agency.

PALPITATIONS

Palpitations are an awareness of the heart beating either due to a change of beat or a heightened awareness of the normal cardiac rate and rhythm.

There are various ways of subdividing arrhythmias, but the most useful in general practice is the distinction between normal and pathological.

Normal (common)
- Increased awareness of the normal heart beat.
- Tachycardia: anxiety feedback loop.
- Menopausal flushing.
- Ventricular ectopics.

Pathological
- Paroxysmal supraventricular tachycardia.
- Atrial fibrillation
  - constant
  - paroxysmal.
- Second- and third-degree heart block.
- Ventricular tachycardia.

Diagnosis

History Ask about:
- Rate and rhythm. (Ask patient to tap on the desk.)
- When the palpitations occur.
- Associated symptoms:
  - faintness/dizziness
  - loss of consciousness (see p. 157)
  - anxiety
  - tingling of the fingers or perioral area (hyperventilation)
  - hot flushes/sweats
  - shortness of breath.
- Exacerbating factors.
- Drug history.
- Cardiovascular history.

Examination
- Anaemia.
- Pulse and BP.
- Thyrotoxic?
- Heart sounds.
- Apex–radial delay (atrial fibrillation).

During attack
- Pulse, BP.
- Signs of heart failure (see p. 154).
- ?MI (see p. 151).

Investigations
- Bloods:
  - FBC
  - C&E
  - thyroid function tests
  - digoxin level.
- ECG:
  - routine
  - during attack.
  (A 24-hour ECG is usually by referral.)

Management

Treatment The following are treatable in general practice.

Non-pathological arrhythmias Reassure (backed up by ECG).

Constant atrial fibrillation If ventricular rate is >100 per minute, and there is no murmur, give digoxin 0.25 mg p.o., then 0.25 mg 12 hours later, and then 0.125 mg daily for 1 week if U&Es are normal. Then assess ventricular rate and adjust dose accordingly.

   Consider anticoagulation with warfarin, unless there are contraindications, in which case give aspirin, 150 mg daily (see p. 366).

Paroxysmal atrial fibrillation Anticoagulate if there are no contraindications; otherwise give aspirin. Digoxin is of no benefit.

Symptomatic supraventricular tachycardia Advise the dive reflex (plunge the face into a sink of cold water)/Valsalva manoeuvre/carotid sinus massage. Stop stimulant intake (coffee, tea, chocolate, cola, etc.).

Emergency treatment of arrhythmias following acute myocardial infarction includes:

- **ventricular tachycardia: lignocaine 100 mg i.v.**
- **sinus bradycardia: atropine 300 μg i.v.**
- **ventricular ectopics: no treatment**
- **ventricular fibrillation: DC shock**
- **asystole: 1:1000 adrenaline 1 ml i.v. and CPR.**

Referral Refer if there is:

- No diagnosis (if symptoms are worrying patient or doctor).
- Atrial fibrillation <60 years of age.
- Atrial flutter.
- Paroxysmal ventricular tachycardia.

- Heart block.
- Associated valvular heart disease.
- Thyrotoxicosis.
- Supraventricular tachycardia not responding to above advice.

RESPIRATORY MEDICINE

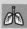

ASTHMA

Asthma is a common chronic disease affecting approximately 5% of adults and 15% of children (see p. 90). It is a disease characterised by increased responsiveness of the airways to a variety of stimuli. The clinical picture is one of wheezing, coughing or shortness of breath, often worse at night. The following is based on the updated British Thoracic Society Guidelines for Asthma published in *Thorax* in 1997.

CHRONIC ASTHMA

Diagnosis

History The suspicion of asthma should be raised if there is a history of chronic recurrent cough or wheeze.

> A diagnosis can be made after more than two episodes of wheeze or cough which respond symptomatically to adequate bronchodilator or prophylactic therapy.

Ask about:

- the duration of symptoms and current treatment
- present symptoms and their effect on lifestyle, e.g. sleep disturbance, time off work or school, effort intolerance
- family history
- atopy
- active and passive smoking
- occupation
- drugs.

Examination/peak flow data

- Examine the chest.
- Measure height (and weight for children).
- Measure the peak flow and calculate the predicted peak flow.
- Prescribe a peak flow meter (if it seems appropriate and the asthma is chronic), available on FP10 (GP10 in Scotland), and teach the use of the peak flow meter and peak flow charts.

In any patient over 12 years old, reversible airways obstruction should ideally be demonstrated via peak flow measurements, either by:

1. a 15% improvement in peak flow 5 minutes after an inhaled bronchodilator

2. a 15% variability in peak flow on a diary kept over a 2-week period when there are no exacerbating factors such as an infection
3. a 15% improvement in peak flow during a trial of high-dose oral steroids.

Management

Advice
- Discuss the disease and the principles of treatment (especially the difference between relief bronchodilators and prophylactic anti-inflammatory treatment).
- Teach an appropriate inhaler technique.
- Discuss a self-management plan, where appropriate.
- Emphasise the need for regular review by the GP or nurse.

Management principles
- Avoid provoking factors, e.g.:
  - smoking (active or passive)
  - house dust mite (cover mattresses and pillows with plastic covers, and minimise carpets, soft furnishings and soft toys, especially in the bedroom)
  - pets
  - drugs: avoid aspirin and NSAIDs.
- Discuss stress as a common exacerbating factor.
- Encourage self-management (see p. 166).

> Advocate the use of prophylactic treatment even with mild asthma (in patients who need a bronchodilator more than once a day). The need for bronchodilators is therefore kept to a minimum.

- Select an appropriate inhaler device. (Aerosol inhalers are always more effective if used with a spacer device.) The use of dry powder, e.g. disks or rotacaps, may be useful for those who find aerosol inhalers difficult to use because of poor coordination.
- Assess inhaler technique regularly, especially if control is poor.
- Treatment should be stepwise (see below), and should be started on the step most appropriate to the severity of the asthma.
- Treatment should be stepped up and down as necessary, depending on the symptoms, the extent of bronchodilator use and the peak flow rate.
- The need for relieving bronchodilators should be kept to a minimum.
- Use short-term oral corticosteroids for severe asthmatic episodes to bring asthma under control.

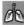

Drug therapy (for older children and adults)

Step one Occasional symptoms: intermittent use of a short-acting bronchodilator to relieve symptoms, e.g. salbutamol 200 µg (two puffs of aerosol) p.r.n.

Step two More frequent symptoms, e.g. if bronchodilator treatment is required more than once a day: regular use of inhaled anti-inflammatory agents, e.g. beclomethasone 100–400 µg (1–4 puffs of beclomethasone 100 aerosol inhalation) b.d. plus short-acting bronchodilators as required.

Step three Worsening symptoms or increasing requirement for bronchodilators: consider sodium cromoglycate 5–10 mg (1–2 puffs) q.d.s. or nedocromil 4 mg (two puffs) b.d. to q.d.s. Alternatively, try regular use of high-dose inhaled steroids, e.g. beclomethasone 500–1000 µg (2–4 puffs of Becloforte aerosol inhalation) b.d. plus short-acting bronchodilators as required. A spacer should always be used. If high-dose inhaled steroids are not tolerated, consider using a long-acting beta agonist inhaler, such as salmeterol 50–100 µg b.d., with a low-dose inhaled steroid.

Step four Worsening symptoms or an increasing requirement for bronchodilators: as above, plus a sequential therapeutic trial of one or more of the following:

- Inhaled long-acting beta agonists, e.g. salmeterol 50–100 µg (2–4 puffs of aerosol) b.d.
- Sustained-release theophylline, e.g. Slo-Phyllin 250–500 mg b.d.
- Inhaled ipratropium 20–40 µg (1–2 puffs of aerosol) 3–4 times daily, or oxitropium 200 µg (two puffs of aerosol) 2–3 times daily.
- Long-acting beta agonist tablets, e.g. Volmax 8 mg b.d.
- High-dose inhaled bronchodilators, e.g. nebulised salbutamol. (Long-term use should be supervised by a chest consultant.)
- Leukotriene receptor antagonist e.g. montelukast 10 mg tablet o.d.

Step five If control is lost at any stage: consider a short course of oral steroids, e.g. prednisolone 30–40 mg mane for 5 days, or until the peak flow has returned to at least 80% of the patient's best ever peak flow. Oral steroids can be stopped abruptly, even after courses of up to 3 weeks, but should not be stopped if the patient is on long-term oral steroids or if the patient's asthma is deteriorating subjectively or objectively.

Referral Refer if:
- asthma remains poorly controlled or if the diagnosis is in doubt
- asthma is thought to involve occupational factors.

Self-management plan Note the patient's predicted or best-ever PEFR, and calculate the 75% and 50% levels. These levels can be marked on a PEFR chart or on the peak flow meter itself. (Remember to recalculate a child's predicted or best-ever peak flow as he/she grows.)

If the patient has an upper respiratory tract infection, is experiencing nocturnal wheezing or a persistent cough, or has a PEFR consistently between 50% and 75% of normal:

- Double the dose of the inhaled steroid for the number of days it takes to return to normal or until the PEFR returns to the previous baseline.
- Continue on this increased dose for the same number of days again. Then return to the maintenance treatment. Use a bronchodilator two puffs 4-hourly, or as appropriate.

If the patient is experiencing shortness of breath with normal activities, is increasing the use of bronchodilators, or has a PEFR which is <50% of normal:

- Double the dose of the inhaled steroids, as above.
- If arrangements have been made to use oral steroids at home:
  – See step 5 (p. 166).
  – The patient should contact the GP within 24 hours.
- If oral steroids are not immediately available, the patient should contact the GP that day.

If the patient is experiencing difficulty speaking, is finding bronchodilators to be ineffective, or has a PEFR which is <30% of normal, he or she should contact the GP urgently, go directly to hospital or call 999.

ACUTE ASTHMA

Many asthma deaths are preventable. Factors include:

- underuse of corticosteroids
- failure of the patient or relatives to appreciate the severity of illness
- failure of the doctor to assess the severity of illness by clinical measurement.

Diagnosis

Examination

Signs of acute severe asthma Seriously consider admission if more than one of the following features are present:

- inability to complete sentences
- a pulse rate of >110 beats per minute
- a respiratory rate of >25 breaths per minute
- a PEFR of <50% of the predicted or best-ever peak flow.

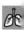

Signs of life-threatening asthma requiring urgent admission • Silent chest
• cyanosis • bradycardia or exhaustion.
Treat as below while awaiting an ambulance.

Management
Lower the threshold for admission if:

- an attack is late in the day
- the patient has had previous severe attacks
- the patient has had recent nocturnal symptoms
- social circumstances are unfavourable.

Treatment
- Treat with a nebulised bronchodilator, e.g. salbutamol 5 mg (2.5 mg in children). If a nebuliser is not available, use salbutamol inhaler via a spacer device, one puff every 30 seconds up to 20 puffs.
- Use oxygen 40–60%, if available.
- Give oral prednisolone 60 mg stat. For children aged <1 year, 1–2 mg/kg; aged 1–5 years, 20 mg stat.
- Consider hydrocortisone 200 mg i.v. in adults.

If the response is good:

- Repeat the nebulised salbutamol 4 hours later. (Leave the nebuliser with the patient.)
- Tell the patient to contact the GP again if the PEFR falls below 50% of its best or the PEFR fails to rise above 75% of its best after nebuliser use.
- Continue oral prednisolone 60 mg daily until recovery is full. For children aged <1 year, 1–2 mg/kg/day; aged 1–5 years, 20 mg/day.

Follow-up
- Assess the adequacy of maintenance treatment.
- Consider prescribing an emergency supply of oral prednisolone for the patient to keep at home.

ASTHMA IN CHILDREN
See page 90.

UPPER RESPIRATORY TRACT INFECTION (URTI)

Upper respiratory tract infections are responsible for about 30% of all GP consultations.

Diagnosis

History Ask about: • sore throat • cough • otalgia • runny nose • blocked nose • dizziness • aches and pains • difficulty swallowing.

Establish the patient's expectations, e.g. antibiotics, sick note, reassurance.

Examination It is usually sufficient to examine the throat, ears and cervical glands. If the patient has a cough, consider examining the chest.

Look particularly for: • quinsy (see p. 224) • tonsillitis (see p. 223) • otitis media (see p. 218) • chest infection (see p. 171).

Management of uncomplicated URTI

- Reassure the patient that the condition is self-limiting and not serious.
- Discourage the use of antibiotics in general. It is often useful to discuss the body's natural immune response.
- Give advice on self-treatments such as paracetamol, soluble aspirin and fluids. Encourage a more self-sufficient approach to minor illness.

Administration

Sick notes are only needed after more than 6 days of continuous absence from work. Form SC2, from the patient's employer, should be used for the first week.

ACUTE COUGH

The commonest presentation in general practice is of an acute URTI. There is a cough, sore throat, a blocked or runny nose or painful cervical glands. Earache or sinus pain may accompany these.

Other symptoms suggest an alternative diagnosis:

Diagnosis

History Ask about:
- The character of the cough:
  - productive
  - dry (asthma, ACE inhibitors).
- Chest pain:
  - pleurisy of pneumonia
  - pulmonary embolus
  - pneumothorax.
- Haemoptysis:
  - pneumonia
  - tuberculosis
  - pulmonary embolus.

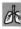

- Purulent sputum:
  - bronchitis
  - bronchiectasis
  - pneumonia.
- Breathlessness:
  - congestive cardiac failure
  - chronic obstructive pulmonary disease.
- Wheeze:
  - asthma
  - chest infection.
- Weight loss:
  - bronchial carcinoma.

Examination Throat, ears, neck, pulse and chest. Pyrexia may be present in carcinoma and pulmonary embolism as well as infection.

Investigations
- CXR, if appropriate.
- ECG in e.g. pulmonary embolus and congestive cardiac failure.

Management
- Simple coughs due to URTI need no specific treatment.
- Lower respiratory tract infections (LRTIs) need antibiotics. Amoxycillin or erythromycin are good first-line antibiotics, with co-amoxiclav or ciprofloxacin for second-line treatment in community-acquired infections.

Referral
- Ill patients with LRTIs should be admitted to hospital.
- Pulmonary embolus: admit the patient to hospital if this is suspected.
- Pneumothorax: admit the patient.
- Bronchial carcinoma: refer to a chest physician.
- Tuberculosis: refer to infectious diseases/chest clinic.
- Congestive cardiac failure (see p. 154).
- Asthma (see p. 164).
- COPD (see p. 175).

Any cough lasting more than 4 weeks falls into the category of chronic cough (see below).

CHRONIC COUGH

A cough that lasts for more than a month can be categorised as a chronic cough.

Diagnosis

Consider the following: • asthma • carcinoma of the bronchus • gastro-oesophageal reflux disease • chronic bronchitis and bronchiectasis • tuberculosis • postnasal drip due to sinusitis.

History Some features make one diagnosis more likely than another. For example, the child with a chronic, dry, nocturnal cough is likely to have asthma, whereas the lifelong heavy smoker aged 65 years with a chronic cough and weight loss is likely to have bronchial carcinoma.

Many adults, however, fall into the category of chronic cough with no obvious associated features.

Examination Chest examination may give some clues, but is often normal in patients with a chronic cough.

Look also for: • clubbing • anaemia • weight loss • maxillary or frontal sinus tenderness • cervical lymphadenopathy • nasal obstruction.

Investigations In suspected asthma, peak flow measurements before and after exercise and also pre- and post-inhalation of salbutamol may give the diagnosis (see p. 164).

A CXR is mandatory in patients aged over 40. Be prepared to repeat this after 6 weeks if the result is normal in patients who are losing weight.

Management

Management is of the underlying condition if this can be diagnosed. Often this is not possible, in which case a stepwise, empirical approach often produces results:

- Give 2 weeks of a broad-spectrum antibiotic, e.g. amoxycillin 500 mg t.d.s. for 5 days.
- If there is no response, give 2 weeks of lansoprazole 15 mg o.d.
- If this fails to cure the cough, try giving 2 weeks of inhaled beclomethasone 400 µg b.d.

If this regimen fails to relieve the symptoms, referral to a chest physician is justified.

> The chronic cough of terminal chest disease can be relieved by pholcodine linctus or morphine.

CHEST INFECTION

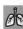

Coughs and colds are the commonest presenting complaints in general practice in the winter and spring months.

Diagnosis

History The commonest presentation is for an URTI to have 'gone onto the chest'.

Ask about:

- cough
- sputum production and colour
- chest pain
- haemoptysis
- breathlessness
- the facial pain of sinusitis
- history of chronic bronchitis or bronchiectasis
- smoking.

Examination Look for:

- Tonsillitis or the pharyngeal mucus of a postnasal drip in sinusitis. Usually the temperature is normal.
- Signs of pneumonia or bronchiectasis (focal crepitations over infected lobes).

Investigations Consider sputum examination and CXR.

Management

- Is the patient unwell? If not, and there are no features in the history or examination to suggest anything other than a simple URTI with a cough, the patient can be reassured that there is nothing seriously wrong. Paracetamol 4-hourly can be advised. The condition should last no more than a week.
- Exacerbations of chronic bronchitis and infective episodes in bronchiectasis require antibiotics. The elderly commonly fall into this group. Oral amoxycillin 500 mg t.d.s. for 1 week is usually sufficient as a first-line choice, with erythromycin or tetracycline as alternatives. If this fails, co-amoxiclav 1 t.d.s. or ciprofloxacin 500 mg b.d. are good second-line choices.
- If pneumonia is suspected, see below.
- Steam inhalation or salbutamol via a metered-dose inhaler can help to loosen sputum.
- Consider asthma in patients with repeated episodes of cough or wheeze (see p. 164).

PNEUMONIA

Pneumonia presents either as a rapidly developing chest infection, or as a consequence of a prior URTI.

Diagnosis

History Ask about:
- cough, which is usually productive
- fever (not always present in the elderly or small children)
- breathlessness
- pleuritic chest pain
- haemoptysis
- vomiting or diarrhoea in children
- falls or confusion in the elderly.

Examination Look for:
- Tachycardia.
- Pyrexia (not always present in the elderly or small children).
- Tachypnoea.
- Coarse crepitations, bronchial breathing and reduced air entry on auscultation of the affected lobe.
- Cyanosis.
- Grunting and intercostal recession, which may be found in small children. Some children may have no chest signs.

Investigations
- CXR if the diagnosis is uncertain.
- Sputum for microscopy and culture if obtainable.
- Dipstick urine for ketones if dehydration is suspected.

Management

 Ill patients should be admitted to hospital, as should all children and the immunocompromised, e.g. diabetics.

- Elderly patients may need admitting for social reasons, e.g. if they live alone.
- The otherwise fit, well-supported adult with no features of systemic toxicity can be started on oral amoxycillin 500 mg t.d.s. or erythromycin 500 mg q.d.s.
- An NSAID, such as ibuprofen, can be useful for pleuritic pain.
- Patients dying of bronchopneumonia (e.g. nursing home residents) may need atropine or hyoscine i.m. for excessive secretions (see p. 331).

 Failure of the pyrexia to respond within 48 hours, or the development of systemic features should prompt admission to hospital.

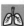

Pneumococcal vaccine See page 200.

HAEMOPTYSIS

The coughing up of blood may vary from slight streaking of phlegm to massive and fatal haemorrhage. A careful history usually allows distinction from haematemesis, although blood swallowed from the upper respiratory tract may be vomited back later.

Diagnosis
Consider the following possible causes:

- URTIs: tonsillitis, sinusitis.
- LRTIs: pneumonia, bronchitis, TB.
- Malignancy: bronchus, larynx, lung secondaries.
- Infarction: pulmonary embolus.

History

> Most cases in general practice involve minor blood-speckling of mucus, produced from the upper respiratory tract due to excessively violent coughing.

Shortness of breath and pleuritic chest pain suggest a pulmonary embolus. A productive cough suggests bronchitis or pneumonia. Chronic cough and weight loss raise the suspicion of a bronchial carcinoma. Known or suspected pulmonary metastases from e.g. a breast primary can present in general practice as haemoptysis.

Examination
- The throat may reveal a possible source of bleeding if the tonsils are inflamed or the fauces injected.
- Chest examination may reveal pneumonia or bronchitis.
- Look for cervical and axillary lymphadenopathy in suspected carcinoma, and weigh the patient if malignancy is suspected.

Investigations
- Send sputum for microscopy and culture if a chest infection is suspected.
- An ECG in pulmonary embolus shows S-waves in lead I and Q-waves and inverted T-waves in lead III.
- A CXR should be considered in TB, carcinoma and pneumonia.

Management

- Manage the underlying disease if a diagnosis is made.
- Haemoptysis can be very distressing. Diazepam orally or i.v. can be useful for acute distress (e.g. in terminal care).

> ⚠ **Admit all cases of haemoptysis heavier than simple streaking of mucus, unless the patient is expected to die, e.g. in palliative care at home.**

- Refer for e.g. diagnostic bronchoscopy if the diagnosis is uncertain.

CHRONIC OBSTRUCTIVE PULMONARY DISEASE (COPD)

COPD is very common in general practice, accounting for 30 000 deaths a year in the UK, and is the sixth leading cause of death worldwide. It is caused mainly by smoking. The following is based on the Royal College of Physicians of Edinburgh consensus statement 2001.

Diagnosis

History COPD should be considered in adults with persistent cough, sputum production or shortness of breath.

Ask about:

- Cough lasting more than one month, or recurrent cough.
- Sputum colour and volume.
- Shortness of breath, which is worse on exertion.
- Smoking (number of packs smoked and number of years as a smoker).
- Any occupational exposure to dust or noxious fumes.
- The effect of the respiratory problems on the patient's daily activities.

Examination

- Look at the chest. Hyperexpansion is common.
- Auscultate for wheeze (common) and signs of infection (also fairly common).
- Clubbing should be absent. Its presence suggests bronchiectasis or lung cancer.
- The heart should not be enlarged and the JVP should not be elevated, unless there is also coexisting heart failure.

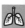

Investigations
- Chest X-ray to help exclude malignancy and heart failure.
- Spirometry. If it is not available in the practice, then referral to a chest clinic for spirometry is strongly recommended. The characteristic feature of COPD is airway obstruction, defined as an FEV_1/VC ratio <70%.
- Reversibility testing: repeat spirometry 5 minutes after a 200 µg dose of inhaled salbutamol. An improvement in FEV_1 of more than 400 ml suggests asthma. Lesser improvements suggest bronchodilators will improve the COPD symptoms.

Referral Consider referral to a chest physician if the patient is:

- under 40 years of age
- a non-smoker
- considerably disabled by dyspnoea
- diagnostically difficult.

Management
Take a stepwise approach to treatment, trialling the following drugs in order. Assess the response by asking the patient what effect there has been on objective measures such as exercise tolerance.

Mild COPD (either mild symptoms, or FEV_1 no less than 50% predicted)
- Short-acting bronchodilator inhaler, such as salbutamol 100 µg, two puffs q.d.s.
- Antimuscarinic, such as ipratropium bromide inhaler 20 µg, two puffs q.d.s., or inhaled tiotropium 18 µg o.d. (especially if there is excessive mucus).

Moderate to severe COPD (FEV_1 <50% predicted, or disabling symptoms)
- Steroid inhaler, such as beclomethasone dipropionate 200–250 µg, two puffs b.d.
- Long-acting beta agonist, such as salmeterol inhaler 25 µg, two puffs b.d.

If none of the above seems to help, consider referral to a chest specialist for consideration for home oxygen therapy.

Prevention

Smoking cessation
This is the only intervention proven to reduce the rate of deterioration in lung function in COPD patients.

- Assess the patient's motivation to quit.
- Offer referral to the practice's smoking cessation lead.
- Consider nicotine replacement therapy and bupropion hydrochloride.
- Hand out a leaflet on smoking cessation and arrange follow-up.

Immunisation
Offer all COPD patients an annual influenza vaccination and pneumococcal vaccination as a one-off.

Acute exacerbation of COPD

An acute exacerbation is a short-term worsening of symptoms, usually caused by infection.

- Increase bronchodilator use.
- Antibiotics, e.g. amoxycillin 250 mg t.d.s. for 1 week, followed by a second-line antibiotic if there has been no response, e.g. co-amoxiclav or ciprofloxacin.
- Oral steroids, especially if there has been a previous good response, or if the patient usually benefits from inhaled steroids. Give prednisolone 30 mg o.d. for 6 days.
- Admit the patient to hospital if:
  - they are considerably disabled by dyspnoea
  - they fail to improve on the above treatment
  - they are unable to cope at home.

INFECTIOUS DISEASES

WHOOPING COUGH

Whooping cough is now rare. After a catarrhal phase, it presents as an increasingly severe and paroxysmal cough. Send a nasopharyngeal swab for diagnosis. A differential white count shows a marked lymphocytosis. The treatment of pertussis is largely symptomatic. Erythromycin given for 10 days prevents spread of the illness. It should also be given to non-immunised child contacts (for pertussis vaccine see p. 195). Admit if symptoms are severe (can cause apnoea in the very young).

Whooping cough is a notifiable disease.

MENINGITIS

There are 2000 cases per year of bacterial meningitis in the UK. Of these, 50% are due to *Neisseria meningitidis*. Viral meningitis is more common.

Diagnosis

History Ask about: • an acute illness of 24–48 hours' duration • fever • headache • photophobia • drowsiness • vomiting • neck stiffness • rash (*N. meningitidis*).

Occasionally, meningitis may develop as a complication of a pre-existing pyrexial illness, such as otitis media, in which case the deterioration will be acute, although the total duration of the illness may be several days.

Examination Look for: • pyrexia • pallor • drowsiness • vomiting • pain on flexing the cervical spine • pain on straight-leg raising • decreased muscle tone in a baby • irritability • a petechial rash which does not blanch on pressure.

Always examine the patient for other causes of pyrexia, e.g. ears, throat, chest.

The early signs of meningitis are those of any pyrexial illness, e.g. pyrexia, irritability, vomiting and lethargy. Always be prepared to re-examine the patient if the condition deteriorates.

Neck pain is more often due to the cervical lymphadenopathy of an upper respiratory tract infection.

Children without meningitis are able to kiss their knees.

Management

Any patient strongly suspected of having meningitis should be seen in hospital as soon as possible, even if there is a possible alternative explanation for the patient's condition, e.g. otitis media.

The vast majority of pyrexial patients will be found on history and examination to have no features of meningitis, and most will have an obvious alternative diagnosis. Treat as appropriate. Take the opportunity to advise the patient or the parents of the features of meningitis.

Close family and school contacts should receive rifampicin 5 mg/kg 12-hourly for 2 days.

> ⚠ **For suspected meningitis give benzylpenicillin i.m./i.v. 600 mg under 2 years of age, 1.2 g over 2 years) immediately, before arranging urgent hospital admission. If allergic to penicillin, give cefotaxime i.m/i.v. 50 mg/kg under 12 years of age, 1 g over 12 years.**

Administration

The hospital should notify the Environmental Health Department.

> Meningitis is a notifiable disease.

SCARLET FEVER

Scarlet fever has become less common over the last 50 years. It is caused by a β-haemolytic *Streptococcus*, group A.

The incubation period is 2–4 days.

Diagnosis

History Ask about: • sore throat • rash • flushed appearance • headache • vomiting.

Examination Look for: • tonsillitis with flecks of pus • tender cervical lymphadenitis • a furred tongue initially, which becomes red and smooth later • a bright pink skin rash with tiny red spots (punctate erythema), which spares the circumoral region • skin peeling, especially on the hands and toes, after a few days.

Investigations Investigations are not indicated, although β-haemolytic *Streptococcus* can be isolated on a throat swab, and elevated ASO titres in blood are found. Usually, by the time the results are available in general practice, the illness is all but over.

Management

Prescribe penicillin V 250 mg q.d.s. orally, or erythromycin if the patient is allergic to penicillin.

Small epidemics of scarlet fever are sometimes seen.

GLANDULAR FEVER

Glandular fever is a common general practice problem, mainly affecting teenagers, but it can present at any age.

The incubation period is usually 7–10 days, occasionally longer.

It can occur either sporadically or in epidemics.

Diagnosis

History Ask about: • sore throat • fever • headaches • tiredness • malaise or anorexia.

These are usually of a short duration, but the condition may present after several weeks of a combination of the above, with prolonged, intermittent symptoms. Upper abdominal pain indicates hepatitis or splenic enlargement.

Examination Look for: • tonsillar enlargement with exudate, which can be difficult to distinguish from bacterial or viral tonsillitis • petechial haemorrhages on the soft palate • posterior cervical lymphadenopathy • hepatosplenomegaly • maculopapular rash.

Investigations

- An FBC and film will show a neutrophil leucocytosis of $10–20 \times 10^9/l$.
- LFTs if jaundice is present.
- A Monospot test will be positive in most cases of glandular fever, especially if taken at least 3 weeks after the start of the illness. False-negative results are common in the first week.

Management

- Advise rest, analgesia and fluids in the acute phase.
- Avoid alcohol.
- Avoid contact sports while the spleen is enlarged.

- Local anaesthetic throat lozenges may be helpful.
- Metronidazole 200 mg t.d.s. may help the oral lesions.
- Prednisolone 30 mg o.d. for 1 week may help if the symptoms are prolonged or severe.
- If the continuing symptoms are dominated by depression, a tricyclic may be of use.
- If lymphadenopathy, fatigue and myalgia persist beyond 3 months, consider postviral fatigue syndrome (see p. 300).

HAND, FOOT AND MOUTH DISEASE

Hand, foot and mouth disease commonly occurs in epidemics. It affects mainly young children and the incubation period is 3–7 days. It is caused by a Coxsackie virus infection.

Diagnosis

History Ask about mild fever and malaise, followed by red spots or vesicles in the mouth and on the lips and buttocks. Milky vesicles also appear on the hands and feet, and these may ulcerate.

Examination Confirms the above. More widespread vesicular lesions suggest chickenpox.

Management

- Symptomatic relief is all that is necessary, using paracetamol and fluids. Benzydamine oral spray is useful for painful oral lesions.
- The illness lasts for 7–10 days.
- Other family members are often affected.

SLAPPED CHEEK (FIFTH DISEASE)

Fifth disease is an infectious upper respiratory illness of small children, which tends to occur in small epidemics.

Diagnosis

History Ask about a mild illness characterised by erythema of the cheeks and accompanied by fever and irritability.

Examination
- Confirm the above.
- Exclude tonsillitis.

Management

There is no specific treatment. Paracetamol helps the fever and irritability.
Associated with increased risk of miscarriage.

 Red cheeks and mild fever may be due to teething in babies.

CHICKENPOX

Chickenpox is a common childhood illness in general practice, occurring
usually in small epidemics.

The incubation period is 2–3 weeks.

After infection with chickenpox, the varicella-zoster virus remains dormant
in dorsal root ganglia. Reactivation causes shingles (see p. 188).

Diagnosis

If the child is seen before the onset of the rash there may be a pyrexia and
irritability. Otherwise the appearance of the rash is diagnostic.

Examination The rash starts with one or two maculopapular spots which are
rapidly joined by many others. Vesicles develop from these as new spots
appear. The rash is very itchy and in children scratch marks can often be seen.
The whole body can be affected, including the palms, soles, oral mucosa and
scalp. In the final stage of the rash, after 5–10 days, the spots scab over.

Complications These are rare: • chickenpox pneumonia (cough, wheeze and
shortness of breath) • encephalomyelitis (signs of meningism).

Management

- Paracetamol and calamine lotion are often all that are needed. Overheating
  tends to make the spots itch more. If impetigo develops in any of the spots,
  use fusidic acid ointment t.d.s. or oral flucloxacillin.
- In adults consider antiviral agent, e.g. aciclovir 800 mg 5 times daily for 7 days.

 **Is the patient immunocompromised? If so, varicella zoster
immunoglobulin may be needed (see p. 202).**

INFLUENZA

Influenza commonly occurs as a winter and spring epidemic.

The incubation period is 24–48 hours.

Diagnosis

History Ask about: • pyrexia • headache • coryza • sore throat • mild photophobia • malaise and myalgia.

Examination Look for: • pyrexia • blocked nose • mild conjunctivitis • red throat and cervical lymphadenopathy.
  Exclude a chest infection, tonsillitis, otitis and meningitis.

> Post-influenza bronchopneumonia is more common in the elderly and infirm and is suspected at the onset of a productive cough, shortness of breath, pleuritic chest pain or prolongation of the fever. Treat with oral flucloxacillin 500 mg q.d.s. for 7 days.

Management

- Rest.
- Analgesic/antipyretic, e.g. aspirin or paracetamol.
- Good fluid intake.
- Reassure patient that they should make a full recovery in 5–6 days.
- Consider prescribing zanamivir inhaler 10 mg b.d. for 5 days when influenza is endemic in the community and if a high-risk patient has presented within 48 hours of the onset of symptoms. High-risk patients are those who are eligible for immunisation against influenza.
- For immunisation against influenza see p. 200.

PNEUMONIA

See page 172.

MALARIA

Malaria is becoming more prevalent in Britain with increased foreign travel. About 2000 cases occur every year in the UK, causing a dozen or so deaths.

Diagnosis

History Ask about:

- Non-specific symptoms, similar to flu, including:
  – fever
  – malaise
  – headache
  – myalgia
  – sweating.
- A history of foreign travel. Visits to equatorial countries within the last year, including airport transfers, are relevant.

 Consider malaria in all patients with a fever after travel to an endemic area.

- The use of antimalarial prophylaxis (see below). A common problem arises when people assume they are immune to malaria, e.g. immigrants visiting relatives in malarious areas.

Examination Examination is often unhelpful in suggesting or confirming the diagnosis. Findings may include fever, jaundice and hepatomegaly.

Investigations Taking blood for a thick blood film for malarial parasites is essential in making the diagnosis. Send 5 ml of blood in a standard haematology tube and request a thick film for malaria. Mark the request urgent and ensure the results are available within 24 hours.

The result should identify the species of parasite.

If the result is negative, but the history strongly suggests the possibility of malaria, repeat the blood film at the height of the fever.

Management

If the diagnosis is confirmed or suspected, discuss the patient with the hospital medical team. An infectious diseases specialist is preferable, if available locally. Most cases are admitted, especially if the infection is due to *Plasmodium falciparum*.

 Malaria is a notifiable disease.

Prevention

There are three important pieces of information to give to travellers about the prevention of malaria:

- Avoid being bitten, e.g. by using mosquito nets and insect repellents and wearing long trousers in the evenings.
- Take the antimalarial tablets as advised, making sure the course is completed (see below).
- Recognise the symptoms of malaria and seek medical help if suspicious: basically, report any febrile illness within 3 months of return from a malarious area.

Drug regimen The choice of antimalarial depends on the area visited, and the advice changes from time to time depending on local resistance of the Anopheles mosquito to chloroquine. For up-to-date advice, either refer to the travel guides published regularly in the free GP magazines or ask the patient to telephone the Medical Advisory Service for Travellers Abroad (MASTA) (see pp. 386 and 387).

> ⚠️ **Whichever drugs are recommended, it is vitally important that they are started 2 weeks prior to travel and continued until 4 weeks after leaving the malarious area.**

Mefloquine should not be taken by patients with depression or other psychiatric disorders, any history of convulsions, or who are pregnant. The alternative antimalarials are less protective against malaria and the patient should reconsider the desirability of travelling to a malarious area.

CONJUNCTIVITIS

See page 234.

DIARRHOEA AND VOMITING

See page 112.

IMPETIGO

See page 126.

COLD SORES

Dry, cracked lips are common, especially during winter, and these can be treated with Vaseline. True herpes simplex (HSV-1) lesions are less common.

Diagnosis

History HSV-1 infection usually affects the lips, tongue, anterior buccal mucosa or nostrils. It is more common in children. It starts with painful ulcers or vesicles, which form singly or in clusters, and is often seen during another upper respiratory tract infection. The vesicles progress to crusts and often become secondarily infected, forming patches of impetigo (see p. 126).

Examination Confirms the above. If the patient presents at the impetigo stage it can be difficult to determine whether or not the underlying lesion is herpetic.

Investigations Herpes virus can be identified by electron microscopy of the vesicular fluid, but in practice this is rarely necessary.

Management
- Symptomatic treatment is often all that is necessary, with the use of analgesics, either orally or topically.
- Acyclovir is very effective in abating an attack of herpes, although its ability to eliminate the virus from the body is less certain.
- Acyclovir cream, 2 g, applied to the lesions five times a day, is usually sufficient if started at the first sign of an attack.
- For lesions inside the mouth, or if the vesicles are widespread in the mouth, valaciclovir tablets can be given 500 mg b.d., or aciclovir suspension 200 mg (5 ml) five times daily over the age of 2 years, 100 mg (2.5 ml) five times daily under age 2 years.
- The total duration of treatment is 5 days.

SHINGLES

The rash of shingles is due to a reactivation of the chickenpox virus.

The incidence of shingles increases with age and is also more common in the immunocompromised.

It is mildly contagious, causing chickenpox, not shingles, in non-immune contacts.

Diagnosis

History The patient experiences tingling, paraesthesia or burning pain in the distribution of a single dermatome (see p. 380). This is followed 24 hours later by the appearance of the rash, starting with erythema, then maculopapular and vesicular lesions and progressing to pustules, crusts and, finally, scars.

Shingles is always unilateral. It is most likely to occur on the trunk, but the face is often affected.

Complications
- Secondary bacterial infection of the vesicles is common, indicated by yellow slough or crusts.
- If the rash is in the trigeminal nerve root distribution, look for spread to the eye or nose.
- Postherpetic neuralgia, i.e. continued pain after the rash has gone, may complicate shingles, especially in the elderly.

Management

Prescribing
- Pain relief is often necessary, e.g. co-proxamol, two tablets 4-hourly.
- Secondary bacterial infection can be treated with fusidic acid ointment t.d.s. or oral flucloxacillin 250 mg q.d.s.
- Postherpetic neuralgia may be improved with amitriptyline 25–75 mg nocte. Alternatively, gabapentin starting at 300 mg daily, increasing to a maximum of 1.8 g daily.
- There is some evidence that zoster-associated pain can be lessened by the use of e.g. oral valaciclovir in patients over 50 years of age presenting within 72 hours of the onset of the rash. The dose is 1 g t.d.s. for 7 days.

Referral
- Arrange for the patient to be seen by an ophthalmologist if the rash involves the eye.
- Admit the patient under the medical or infectious diseases team if the rash becomes extensive.

BOILS

The boil, or furuncle, is a common skin infection, occurring even in people with adequate hygiene.

Diagnosis

History A spot, almost anywhere on the body, becomes painful and inflamed. This progresses to a tense, swollen, erythematous lump. If left, the boil eventually points (forms a head) and either regresses or discharges its contents.

Boils often come in crops, one after another, and tend to be recurrent.

Examination Look for: • the above features • lymphangitis from the boil to the regional lymph nodes • lymphadenopathy.

Investigations
- A swab of the pus, if the boil is discharging, can guide antibiotic choice.
- For recurrent boils, take nasal swabs to check for *Staphylococcus aureus*, in case the patient is a carrier. Exclude diabetes.

Management
- Analgesia is often all that is required.
- Dress with magnesium sulphate paste under an absorbent dressing if the boil looks ready to discharge.
- Prescribe flucloxacillin 250 mg q.d.s. for 5 days if the surrounding skin is erythematous or if lymphangitis is present.
- If the boil is very tense and painful, relief may be gained by incising it through its pointing head with the tip of a scalpel blade, after spraying the boil with e.g. ethyl chloride. The boil can be gently squeezed to massage pus out and a dry dressing applied.
- If the patient is found to be a carrier of *Staphylococcus*, prescribe Naseptin cream, oral flucloxacillin and an antiseptic shower soap for 2 weeks.

HEPATITIS

Hepatitis A is the most common form of hepatitis seen in general practice in the UK. The incubation period is about 1 month. Infection spreads by the faecal–oral route, or by ingestion of infected food.

Hepatitis B is acquired parenterally, e.g. by blood transfusion, needlestick injury or sexually.

Prior to 1991, hepatitis C in the UK was usually caused by infected blood transfusion. Since the introduction of screening blood donors, the commonest cause of hepatitis C has been intravenous drug misuse.

Diagnosis

History Patients may be asymptomatic, especially in hepatitis A. Infection with hepatitis B and C viruses is also usually asymptomatic, except in intravenous drug users, in whom 30% of hepatitis B infections are associated with jaundice

By the age of 50 about 50% of the population in the UK is immune to hepatitis A.

Early symptoms of hepatitis
These can include:

- malaise
- nausea
- mild fever
- headache
- a distaste for cigarettes
- anorexia and diarrhoea
- upper abdominal pain
- pale stools and dark urine, which herald the onset of jaundice
- skin rashes and arthralgia, which can occur in hepatitis B.

Examination
- Jaundice is most evident in the sclerae.
- Lymphadenopathy and splenomegaly may be present.
- The liver is usually tender but not palpable.
- The urine tests positive for bilirubin, even in anicteric cases.

Investigations
- LFTs: show a raised AST and bilirubin.
- FBC: shows a lymphocytosis.
- Hepatitis viral screen: anti-HAV IgM shows a rising titre over 7–10 days in acute hepatitis A.
- Prothrombin time should remain normal. (A rising prothrombin time indicates hepatic failure.)
- Hepatitis B surface antigen is diagnostic of acute hepatitis B. Five to ten per cent of patients go on to develop chronic hepatitis. In these the surface antigen remains positive. If they are also e-antigen positive, they remain highly infectious.
- Antibodies to hepatitis C appear relatively late in the course of the disease. If clinical suspicion is high, test for hepatitis C virus RNA to establish the diagnosis.

Management
- No specific treatment is needed for hepatitis A or B.
- Bed rest is initially advisable, with simple analgesics for muscle or abdominal pains.
- The acute illness usually resolves in 3–6 weeks.
- A full, well-balanced diet and adequate fluid intake are recommended.
- Monitor for signs of fulminant hepatic failure (confusion, disordered LFTs).
- In hepatitis B and C warn the patient of spread to sexual contacts.
- Offer hepatitis B immunisation to family members and sexual contacts.

- Patients testing positive for hepatitis C should be referred for consideration for interferon α to reduce the risk of chronic infection.
- In acute hepatitis B check for hepatitis B surface antigen at 3 months. Only about 5–10% remain positive in the UK.
- All such patients should be referred for expert follow-up.
- For immunisation see page 201.

> General malaise for 2–3 months is common. Alcohol should be avoided for 6 months. Oral contraceptives can be resumed after clinical and biochemical recovery.

> The viral causes of hepatitis are notifiable diseases. Isolation is not necessary, but good personal hygiene is advisable to prevent the spread of infection. Children can return to school as soon as clinical recovery allows.

HIV/AIDS

Over 20 000 people in the UK are known to be HIV-positive, with about 3000 new cases per year. All persons who are sexually active should be advised on the prevention of HIV and AIDS. Safe- and low-risk sex should be promoted (see p. 2).

Increasing numbers of patients are requesting HIV testing in the wake of a growing public awareness of the disease and its risk factors. HIV testing is only performed with the patient's consent.

> Not all GPs feel able to provide appropriate counselling. Genitourinary medicine clinics can.

The test must be delayed until at least 3 months after the at-risk exposure, as this is considered to be the time taken for seroconversion to occur.

Pre-test counselling
- Take a brief history to ascertain why the patient wants the test and his or her likely risk. Risk factors include:
  - sexual contact with a known HIV-positive person
  - intravenous drug use

- homosexual contact
- needlestick injury
- sex with men or women in high-risk countries, e.g. Thailand and sub-Saharan Africa
- sex with prostitutes.
- Ask the patient to consider the implications of a positive result.
- Give advice on safe sex and needle use, if appropriate.
- Arrange another appointment for the patient to be told the result and make sure this is not a Friday, as counselling for newly diagnosed HIV-positive patients may be difficult to organise over a weekend.

The follow-up appointment

- It is probably best not to give results by telephone, as the opportunity for post-test counselling may be lost.
- If the result is negative, the patient did not have antibodies to HIV at the time of the test. A further test is indicated if there has been continued possible exposure to the virus.
- Reiterate the advice on safe sex and needle use.
- If the result is positive, allow time for the bad news to sink in and be prepared for extremes of emotion. Answer questions honestly and as fully as possible. Offer hope: most HIV-positive people remain asymptomatic for many years, patients have now survived over 10 years with HIV, and new drugs are being developed and used which delay the progression of the disease. (See: breaking bad news, p. 322.)
- Inform the patient that he or she will be followed up in the genitourinary clinic and of the availability of expert HIV counsellors at such clinics. Arrange the referral by telephone and give the patient an appointment time. It should be possible to do this before seeing the patient once you have sight of the positive result.
- Offer the patient a follow-up appointment after 24–48 hours to answer further questions.

HIV-positive patients

Patients with HIV-positive status should be followed up regularly in a department of genitourinary medicine or a specialist HIV clinic.

The GP should consider the HIV-positive patient to be immuno-compromised, i.e. any pyrexial illness should be treated seriously. Patients with a low T4 count should be admitted.

Chest infections may be due to *Pneumocystis carinii*. Tuberculosis is also not uncommon.

Close liaison with the patient's consultant is essential. There is a greater need to consider confidentiality as a sensitive issue in many cases of HIV disease.

IMMUNISATIONS

Childhood immunisations

Every effort should be made to immunise all children, even if they are older than the recommended age range. A minor non-febrile illness should not be a reason for delaying vaccination.

The schedule for routine immunisation is as shown in the table below.

Neonates should receive BCG if at high risk (see p. 199) and/or hepatitis B vaccine if the mother is a carrier (see p. 201).

Routine childhood immunisations		
Vaccine	**Age**	**Comment**
DTP, polio, Hib and meningitis C, 1st dose	2 months	Primary course
DTP, polio, Hib and meningitis C, 2nd dose	3 months	
DTP, polio, Hib and meningitis C, 3rd dose	4 months	
Measles/mumps/rubella (MMR)	12–15 months	Can be given at any age over 12 months
Booster diphtheria/tetanus, acellular pertussis and polio, and MMR (2nd dose)*	3–5 years	3 years after completion of primary course
BCG	10–14 years	For tuberculin-negative children
Booster diphtheria (low dose)/tetanus and polio*	13–18 years	
DTP, Diphtheria/tetanus/pertussis (whole cell). *Note that no booster dose of Hib or meningitis C is required after the primary course.		

Adult vaccinations

Adults should receive the following vaccines:

- Non-pregnant women who are seronegative for rubella: rubella.
- Previously unimmunised individuals: polio, tetanus, diphtheria.
- Individuals in high-risk groups: hepatitis B, hepatitis A, influenza, pneumococcal vaccine.

Live vaccines

These include the following: • polio • rubella • measles • mumps • BCG • yellow fever.

Live vaccines should not be given to:

- Pregnant women. (The risk is theoretical, so live vaccine may be given if there is a significant risk of exposure.)

- The immunocompromised (e.g. treatment with high-dose corticosteroids (prednisolone 40 mg per day for 1 week or more, in adults; 2 mg/kg per day in children) within the last 3 months, malignancy of the reticuloendothelial system, treatment with radiotherapy).

HIV-positive patients may be given most live vaccines, but should *not* be given BCG or yellow fever.

When two live vaccines are required, they should be given either simultaneously at different sites or with an interval of at least 3 weeks. If time constraints make this impossible, it is better to give them within 3 weeks of each other than to omit them.

Immunoglobulin may interfere with the development of active immunity from live vaccines. Live vaccines should therefore be given at least 3 weeks before or 3 months after immunoglobulin. If time constraints make this impossible, this advice may have to be ignored.

Passive immunisation

Normal immunoglobulin is available for prophylaxis of measles and hepatitis A. Specific immunoglobulins are available for tetanus, hepatitis B, rabies and varicella-zoster.

For more detailed information on immunisations, refer to *Immunisation against Infectious Diseases*, published by HMSO and distributed free to every surgery.

PERTUSSIS VACCINE

A reinforcing dose of acellular pertussis vaccine is necessary after the primary course of whole cell pertussis and is given between 3 and 5 years of age.

Adverse reactions

- Local swelling and redness, fever and malaise are common.
- There is no conclusive evidence to show that brain damage has ever been caused by the vaccine; however, the vaccine may very rarely be associated with an acute severe neurological illness in previously normal children, from which recovery is full.

Contraindications

- Postpone immunisation if:
  - The child is suffering from an acute febrile illness.
  - There is an evolving neurological problem. Immunisation should be deferred until the condition is stable.
- Do not vaccinate children who have had a severe local or general reaction to a preceding dose:
  - A severe local reaction is swelling and induration involving most of the injected part of the limb.
  - A severe general reaction is a fever of >39.5°C, inconsolable screaming for >4 hours, or any more severe reaction.

- If there is a personal or family history of febrile convulsions, there is an increased risk of these occurring after pertussis immunisation. Immunisation *should* be given, but advice on fever prevention should be given at the time of vaccination.

DIPHTHERIA VACCINE

Immunisation is recommended for:

- All children.
- All non-immune adults.
- All contacts. Immune contacts require a booster. Non-immune contacts require a full course of three doses at monthly intervals and a prophylactic course of erythromycin.
- Travel, if appropriate.

The primary course is given routinely together with tetanus and pertussis as part of the triple vaccine at 2, 3 and 4 months. A booster is given at 3–5 years together with tetanus and pertussis. A further reinforcing dose is now recommended at school-leaving (low-dose diphtheria, usually given with tetanus vaccine).

Low-dose diphtheria vaccine should be used in patients over 10 years because of the possibility of a serious reaction in a patient who is already immune.

The Schick test is used to ensure immunity to diphtheria in those who may be exposed to diphtheria in the course of their work.

Contraindications

- Postpone immunisation if the child is suffering from an acute febrile illness.
- Do not vaccinate if there has been a severe local or general reaction to a preceding dose. (Reactions to the pertussis or tetanus components of the triple vaccine are more likely.)

TETANUS VACCINE

Children

Tetanus is given as part of the triple vaccine at 2, 3 and 4 months of age and reinforced at ages 3–5 and 13–18 years. If a course is interrupted it may be resumed; there is no need to start again.

Adults

Elderly women are at highest risk of the disease.

Previously unimmunised adults should be given primary immunisation (three doses with intervals of 1 month between each dose). They will require two booster doses at 10-year intervals. After five doses, as above, immunity is likely to be lifelong.

A tetanus-prone wound

This is any wound or burn sustained more than 6 hours before surgical treatment that shows one of the following:

- a significant degree of devitalised tissue
- a puncture-type wound
- contact with soil or manure
- evidence of sepsis.

Patients with a tetanus-prone wound who are not immunised should receive a primary course. Those who had their last booster >10 years ago should receive a booster. Both groups should be given a dose of tetanus immunoglobulin.

Contraindications
- An acute febrile illness.
- Adverse reaction to a previous dose.

HAEMOPHILUS INFLUENZA B (HIB) VACCINE

Hib vaccine is recommended for all babies from 2 months, together with the triple vaccine and polio. The primary course consists of three doses with an interval of 1 month between each dose. No booster doses are necessary.

Unimmunised children between 13 and 48 months should be given a single injection of Hib vaccine only, as they are at lower risk of disease. Routine immunisation is not recommended after age 4 years.

Unimmunised household contacts of Hib under the age of 4 years should receive Hib vaccine. Independently of immunisation, rifampicin prophylaxis should be given.

POLIO VACCINE

Oral polio vaccine is recommended for all infants from 2 months of age. The primary course consists of three separate doses with intervals of 1 month between each dose, given at the same time as DTP and Hib vaccines. Two booster doses are given:

- before starting school at age 4.5 years
- before leaving school at age 13–18 years.

The primary immunisation of adults consists of three doses of oral polio vaccine at intervals of 4 weeks. Booster doses for adults are unnecessary unless they are at special risk, e.g. travellers to epidemic or endemic areas, contacts of polio.

Faecal excretion of vaccine virus can last up to 6 weeks, so unimmunised parents should be immunised at the same time as their child. Contacts of a recently immunised baby should be advised to wash their hands carefully after changing the baby's nappies.

Contraindications
- An acute febrile illness.
- Vomiting or diarrhoea.
- Immunosuppression.
- Reticuloendothelial system malignancy.
- Extreme sensitivity to penicillin, streptomycin, neomycin or polymyxin.
- As for all live vaccines (see p. 194).

MEASLES/MUMPS/RUBELLA VACCINE

MMR is recommended for all children aged 12–15 months. A second dose is given to preschool children at the age of 3–5 years. It should be given despite a previous history of measles, mumps or rubella. MMR can be given to children of any age whose parents request it, and should be encouraged, especially for children who have never been immunised against measles. All children aged under 5 years should receive two doses at least 3 months apart. It can also be given to non-immune adults.

MMR vaccine is used to protect non-immune measles contacts, and must be given within 3 days of exposure. Immunoglobulin is given for contacts in whom vaccine is contraindicated.

Side-effects
- Malaise, fever and/or a rash may occur 1 week after immunisation.
- Febrile convulsions occur in 1:1000 children at the same stage. Parotid swelling occurs in 1:100 children in the third week.
- Mumps meningoencephalitis occurs in 1:300 000 children.
- There is no convincing scientific evidence that the MMR vaccine causes Crohn's disease or autism

Contraindications
- Acute febrile illness.
- Immunosuppression.
- Allergy to neomycin, kanamycin or polymyxin.
- As for other live vaccines (see p. 194).
- MMR should not be given within 3 months of an injection of immunoglobulin.
- Pregnancy.
- Women who have been given MMR should avoid pregnancy for 1 month.

MUMPS VACCINE

Adults requiring mumps protection may be given either MMR or mumps vaccine. There is no available protection for contacts.

RUBELLA VACCINE

Rubella is part of the MMR vaccine given at 12–15 months and again at 3–5 years of age. All girls aged between 10 and 14 years should be given a single dose of rubella vaccine unless there is documented evidence of MMR having been previously given.

- All women of child-bearing age should be screened for rubella antibodies.
- Non-immune women should receive a single dose of rubella vaccine unless they are pregnant. An LMP of <4 weeks previously excludes pregnancy.
- Advise women against pregnancy for 1 month after immunisation (see p. 22).
- Seronegative pregnant women should be immunised after pregnancy.
- There is no adequate protection for contacts.

Contraindications
As for MMR.

BCG VACCINE

BCG is recommended for the following groups, provided the tuberculin skin test is negative.

- Those at normal risk:
  - all children aged 10–14 years, according to local policy
  - all students, according to local policy
  - babies, children or adults where the parents or the individuals themselves request BCG immunisation.
- Those at higher risk:
  - health service and veterinary staff
  - contacts of cases of active respiratory tuberculosis
  - immigrants from countries with a high prevalence of tuberculosis, and their children, wherever born
  - travellers to high-prevalence areas for >1 month.

BCG immunisation and tuberculin skin-testing are organised at local chest clinics.

Contraindications
- Positive tuberculin skin test.
- Pyrexia.
- Immunosuppression.
- Malignancy of the reticuloendothelial system.
- Pregnancy.
- Those who are HIV-positive.
- As for other live vaccines (see p. 194).

The tuberculin skin test (Mantoux or Heaf)

A tuberculin skin test must be carried out before BCG immunisation (except in infants up to 3 months old, who may be immunised without a prior test). A positive test implies past infection or past successful immunisation and BCG should not then be given.

INFLUENZA VACCINE

Influenza vaccine is recommended for everyone aged over 65 years, and all adults and children with any of the following:

- Chronic respiratory disease, including asthma.
- Chronic heart disease.
- Chronic renal failure.
- Diabetes mellitus and other endocrine disorders.
- Immunosuppression, including asplenia.
- It is also recommended for residents of nursing homes, old people's homes and other long-stay establishments.

Adults require one injection annually. Children require a primary course of two injections 4–6 weeks apart, and then annual injections. The ideal time for immunisation is late October/early November.

Warn patients that they will still be susceptible to colds and sore throats due to other viruses. Patients being given influenza vaccine should be considered for pneumococcal vaccine (see below).

Contraindications

- Anaphylactic egg allergy.
- Pregnancy.

PNEUMOCOCCAL VACCINE

Pneumococcal vaccination should be considered for all those aged >2 years for whom the risk of contracting pneumococcal pneumonia is unusually high or dangerous, i.e. those with: • asplenia • homozygous sickle cell disease • immunosuppression • chronic renal failure (or nephrotic syndrome), heart, lung or liver disease • diabetes mellitus.

A single dose only is needed.

Pneumococcal vaccine may be given with influenza vaccine at a different site. Reimmunisation is only considered in those at greatest risk, e.g. asplenia or nephrotic syndrome, after 5–10 years.

Contraindications

- Acute infection.
- Pregnancy.
- Within 3 years of a previous dose of pneumococcal vaccine.

HEPATITIS A VACCINE

Hepatitis A vaccine is recommended for:

- Travellers: for those who frequently visit areas of high/moderately high risk, such as Africa or the Far East, or for those staying in such areas for >3 months. Testing for antibodies to hepatitis A is advised prior to immunisation in those who are already likely to be immune:
  - those >50 years old
  - those born in areas of high hepatitis A virus endemicity
  - those with a history of jaundice.
- Occupational exposure, e.g. sewage workers.
- Patients with chronic liver disease.
- Haemophiliacs.
- Homosexuals whose sexual behaviour is likely to put them at high risk.
- Community outbreaks.

A single dose confers immunity for 1 year. A booster dose at 6–12 months extends immunity for up to 10 years.

Give children under 15 years old Havrix Junior.

Immunoglobulin gives short-term protection against hepatitis A to travellers (if appropriate) and to contacts. It can be given at the same time as hepatitis A vaccine if protection is required within 10 days of the first dose of hepatitis A vaccine. One injection only is necessary. There are two dosage levels. Use the higher dose for contacts and for extended protection (i.e. those travelling abroad for 3–5 months). For information on live vaccines see page 194.

Contraindications
- Pyrexia.
- Pregnancy. (It should not be given unless there is a definite risk of infection.)

HEPATITIS B VACCINE

Hepatitis B vaccination is recommended in those at risk of contracting the virus, e.g. healthcare workers, staff and residents of homes for those with severe learning difficulties, drug abusers, those who change sexual partners frequently, prisoners, chronic renal disease patients, haemophiliacs.

Vaccination is unnecessary in those who are hepatitis B surface antigen positive.

- Three doses at 0, 1 and 6-month intervals are given.
- Check the antibody levels 3–4 months after the last dose. Non-responders should receive a fourth dose.
- A single booster dose 5 years after the primary course may be sufficient to maintain immunity.

Specific hepatitis B immunoglobulin can be given for post-exposure prophylaxis (passive protection), e.g. after accidental inoculation. It should be given within 48 hours of exposure, and is normally used in combination with hepatitis B vaccine.

MENINGOCOCCAL VACCINE

The major cause of meningococcal disease in the UK is group B, against which there is no available vaccine. There are two vaccines against the other types of bacterial meningitis: meningitis C vaccine and the combined meningitis A and C vaccine.

Meningitis C vaccine is recommended for:

- babies at ages 2, 3 and 4 months, along with DTP–Hib and polio vaccines
- previously unimmunised adults aged ≤ 24 years – single dose.

Meningitis A and C vaccination is recommended for:

- close contacts of cases of group A or group C meningitis, who should be given meningococcal vaccine in addition to chemoprophylaxis
- control of local outbreaks in close communities
- for travellers, as appropriate, even if they have already received meningitis C vaccine.

The vaccine is effective for 3 years.

Contraindications
- Febrile illness.
- A severe previous reaction.
- Pregnancy.

CHICKENPOX AND HERPES ZOSTER IMMUNISATION

Passive immunisation only is available in the form of human varicella-zoster immunoglobulin. Varicella-zoster immunoglobulin is recommended for contacts of chickenpox or herpes zoster in the following groups:

- Those who are immunosuppressed.
- Those with debilitating disease.
- Non-immune pregnant women. Varicella-zoster immunoglobulin will not prevent congenital varicella syndrome, but it may attenuate the disease in pregnant women.
- Infants up to 4 weeks old:
  - whose mothers develop chickenpox from 7 days before to 1 month after delivery
  - who are in contact with chickenpox or zoster when their mother has no antibody on testing.

The supply of varicella-zoster immunoglobulin is limited by the availability of suitable donors.

Aciclovir should be used in the treatment of severe disease (see p. 184).

RABIES VACCINE

Pre-exposure prophylaxis

This should be offered to:

- anyone who, by the nature of their work, is likely to have contact with rabies
- travellers to high-risk areas where medical treatment might not be immediately available.

Rabies vaccine is only free on the NHS for the first category of patient.

The course consists of three doses at days 0, 7 and 28. Give booster doses at 2–3-year intervals to those at continued risk.

Post-exposure treatment

- Ask about the rabies risk in the country concerned.
- Cleanse the wound thoroughly.
- Give:
  - Six doses of rabies vaccine on days 0, 3, 7, 14, 30 and 90. If the biting animal is symptom-free after 10 days of observation, stop treatment.
  - Rabies-specific immunoglobulin.

Contraindications

There are no absolute contraindications to rabies vaccine.

CHOLERA VACCINE

Cholera vaccination should not be required of any traveller. However, local officials sometimes require it, and one injection is sufficient to provide a certificate.

Contraindications

- Acute febrile illness.
- Hypersensitivity to previous dose.
- Pregnancy.

TYPHOID VACCINE

Give typhoid vaccine to travellers, if appropriate.

Vi polysaccharide vaccine A polysaccharide vaccine can be given as a single dose only, with a booster dose every 3 years on continued exposure.

Oral typhoid vaccine A live attenuated vaccine requires three doses of one capsule on alternate days. Protection lasts for 1–3 years.

Side-effects
- Local reactions to polysaccharide vaccine are usually mild, and systemic reactions are uncommon.

Contraindications
- Acute febrile illness.
- Severe reaction to previous dose.
- Pregnancy.

YELLOW FEVER VACCINE

Yellow fever vaccine is recommended for:

- laboratory workers handling infected material
- persons aged 9 months and over, travelling through or living in infected areas
- travellers requiring an International Certificate of Vaccination for entry into a country.

A single dose confers immunity for 10 years. The vaccine can only be given at yellow fever vaccination centres.

Precautions against mosquito bites should be taken.

Adverse reactions
- Mild flu-like symptoms in 5–10% of recipients 5–10 days after immunisation.
- Rarely, anaphylaxis and encephalitis have been reported.

Contraindications
- The usual contraindications to a live vaccine (see p. 194).
- Those who are hypersensitive to neomycin or polymyxin or who have had an anaphylactic reaction to egg.
- HIV-positive individuals.

JAPANESE B ENCEPHALITIS VACCINE

Japanese B encephalitis is a mosquito-borne viral encephalitis.

Vaccination is recommended for travellers who will be staying for a month or longer in endemic areas, especially if travel will include rural areas.

The vaccine schedule is three doses on days 0, 7–14 and 28. Full immunity takes up to 1 month to develop. A booster is recommended after 2 years, if at risk. The vaccine must be given on a named-patient basis, as it is unlicensed in the UK. Precautions against mosquito bites should be taken.

Adverse reactions
- Local reaction.
- Allergic reactions, and occasionally angioneurotic oedema occurring within minutes or up to 2 weeks after receiving the vaccine.

Contraindications
- Fever.
- History of anaphylactic hypersensitivity.
- Pregnancy.
- Cardiac, renal or hepatic disorders and generalised malignancy.

TICK-BORNE ENCEPHALITIS VACCINE

This is recommended for walkers and campers in late spring and summer, in forested areas of central and eastern Europe and Scandinavia.

Two doses are given 4–12 weeks apart, giving protection for 1 year. The vaccine is available on a named-patient basis.

Protection is afforded by covering arms, tucking long trousers into socks and using insect repellent on outer clothing.

Adverse reactions
- Very rarely, local and flu-like reactions occur.
- Rarely, neurological symptoms have occurred.

Contraindications
Allergy to egg protein.

MALARIA

See page 185.

ADMINISTRATION

- Make a record of the immunisation in a prominent or dedicated part of the patient's clinical file.

PYREXIA OF UNKNOWN ORIGIN (PUO)

In theory, a PUO is a pyrexia greater than 38°C, lasting more than 3 weeks, with no known cause after extensive investigation.

In general practice, thorough investigation is not possible. Many patients present with a temperature, and in some of these the cause will not be found with any great certainty. It is, however, rare in general practice for a genuine pyrexia to last more than 2 weeks.

History Ask about:
- The method of recording the temperature. Patients may say they have a raised temperature when they actually mean they feel hot/sweaty/flushed. Advise the use of an oral thermometer if in doubt.

- Medication: drugs which can cause pyrexia include:
  - antibiotics
  - antituberculous drugs
  - anticonvulsants
  - propylthiouracil
  - quinidine
  - procainamide.
- Other symptoms: rash, myalgia, weight loss, pain, cough.
- Contact with infectious disease.
- Past medical history: e.g. malignancies, HIV.
- Animal contact: parrots (psittacosis).
- Travel, especially to malarious areas.

Examination Look for:
- Clubbing, splinter haemorrhages, joint effusions, rashes.
- Ear, nose and throat infections.
- Cervical lymphadenopathy.
- Chest infection.
- Heart murmurs.
- Organomegaly.

Investigations
- FBC: infection, lymphoma, leukaemia.
- ESR: infections, malignancies, temporal arteritis.
- LFT: malignancies, hepatitis.
- Urine: infection, renal cancers.
- Stool: tropical infection, *Clostridium difficile*.
- CXR: TB, sarcoid, lymphoma, psittacosis, metastases.

Management

 Most persistent fevers can be diagnosed with a thorough history, examination and the above simple investigations. In the absence of a diagnosis, referral to an infectious diseases specialist is warranted once the pyrexia has lasted more than 4 weeks.

The use of antibiotics 'blind' is to be avoided in prolonged pyrexia. Refer for diagnosis first.

WEIL'S DISEASE

Weil's disease is the rare form of leptospirosis with jaundice that is usually caught from infected rat's urine and therefore affects mainly sewage workers, water board workers and people who swim in contaminated rivers.

History Ask about:
- Exposure to potentially contaminated water in the preceding 7–21 days.
- Abrupt onset of headache, severe muscular aches, chills and fever up to 39°C.
- Initial symptoms for 4–9 days followed by a recurrence of symptoms after a few days of relief.
- Jaundice occurs on day 3–6 in Weil's disease.

Examination Look for:
- conjunctival redness
- jaundice
- haemorrhages
- anaemia
- haematuria.

Investigations
- FBC: anaemia, neutrophil leucocytosis.
- LFT: raised bilirubin.
- Serology: acute (days 2–4) and convalescent (week 3–4) for antibodies to leptospires.
- Blood cultures: for leptospires early in the disease, if suspected.

Management

> Mild cases without jaundice can be confused with flu-like illnesses but make a full recovery anyway.

Jaundiced patients with a history of a biphasic febrile illness, headache, severe muscle pains and possible exposure to rat's urine should be admitted for investigation and intravenous antibiotic treatment of suspected Weil's disease.

The mortality in jaundiced patients is 10%.

LYME DISEASE

Lyme disease is a flu-like illness characterised by the rash of erythema migrans. It is caused by the spirochete *Borrelia burgdorferi*, and is transmitted by tick bite, usually from deer ticks in areas such as the New Forest.

History Ask about:
- A large, red insect bite, usually on the thigh, trunk or axilla, often followed by smaller red marks around the initial area.
- A severe headache.
- Myalgia, malaise, fatigue.
- Travel in an endemic area – New Forest, American North East.
- History of tick bite.

Examination Look for:
- A large red, raised ring lesion with central clearing (the eschar).
- Similar smaller surrounding lesions which come and go (migrans).
- Later in the illness there may be signs of arthritis.

Investigations Acute and convalescent anti-spirochetal antibodies confirm the diagnosis, but treatment can begin if the condition is suspected on clinical grounds.

Management
- Discuss the case with the infectious diseases department.
- Outpatient treatment is usually possible, with oral antibiotics such as amoxicillin 500 mg t.d.s. for 10–14 days, or doxycycline 100 mg b.d. for 10–14 days.
- Most features of the disease respond well, especially if treated early.
- Complications include arthritis, Bell's palsy, heart block and lymphocytic meningitis. These are rare.

MEASLES

Measles is now uncommon in Britain due to the high uptake of the MMR vaccine and, previously, measles vaccines. Measles is more common towards the end of the year.

The incubation period is 2 weeks.

Diagnosis

History and examination Upper respiratory features predominate initially, with conjunctivitis, rhinitis, otitis media and fever as well as Koplik's spots on the buccal mucosa (discrete small, white spots). This is followed 24–48 hours later by the appearance of the dusky pink macular rash, initially on the face and spreading peripherally.

Uncomplicated measles lasts 7–10 days.

Investigation The diagnosis may be confimed by a rising IgM titre between acute and convalescent sera.

Complications
- Bacterial otitis media.
- Bronchopneumonia.
- Purulent conjunctivitis.
- Giant cell pneumonitis (rare).
- Allergic encephalomyelitis (1:6000 cases).
- Subacute sclerosing panencephalitis (1:1 000 000 cases).

Management
- There is no specific treatment for uncomplicated measles.
- Secondary bacterial infections should respond to the appropriate antibiotic.
- Human normal immunoglobulin is advisable for immunocompromised patients.
- For childhood immunisation against measles, see p. 198.

 Measles is a notifiable disease.

MUMPS

Mumps is becoming increasingly rare following the introduction of the MMR vaccine. Mumps is most common in school-age children and young adults.

The incubation period is 18–21 days.

Diagnosis

History Ask about fever and malaise for 1 or 2 days, followed by parotid gland swelling and pain.

Examination The parotid gland swelling of mumps makes the angle of the jaw impalpable, helping to distinguish it from cervical or submandibular lymphadenopathy.

Investigation Send saliva sample, during parotitis, for detection of virus.

Complications
- Orchitis affects 1 in 4 males who contract the disease after puberty.
- Abdominal pain, usually due to pancreatitis or oophoritis.
- Acute lymphocytic meningitis.

Management
- Most cases involve only a straightforward parotitis. There is no specific treatment for this other than pain and temperature control using paracetamol.

- Orchitis may respond to prednisolone 40 mg o.d. in adults for 4 days.
- Abdominal pain may be managed conservatively at home with analgesia, if the patient remains systemically well.
- In most cases the illness lasts only 2–3 days.
- For childhood immunisation against mumps, see p. 198.

Mumps meningitis must be managed in hospital, even though the treatment is conservative, as a lumbar puncture is required to rule out the possibility of bacterial meningitis.

Mumps is a notifiable disease.

RUBELLA

Rubella is becoming increasingly rare with the widespread use of the MMR vaccine.

The incubation period is 2.5–3 weeks.

Diagnosis

History Rubella is often a mild illness characterised by conjunctival suffusion and rhinitis, followed, after 24 hours, by a discrete, light pink maculopapular rash.

Examination Examination confirms the features in the history. Also present are enlarged lymph nodes in the postauricular and suboccipital groups.

Investigations Investigations are unnecessary except in pregnant women without proven immunity who are in contact with a suspicious rash. Send 10 ml of clotted blood to the virology laboratory for haemagglutination and IgM titres. Repeat serology may be requested after 10 days.

Differential diagnosis The commonest confusion is with roseola infantum and non-specific viral rashes. Rubella is unusual without a certain amount of lymphadenopathy, which is often lacking in the non-specific illnesses.

Complications Complications are very unusual. Joint pain is probably the most common.

Management
- Symptomatic treatment is usually all that is required. The rash should last no longer than 5 days.

- Refer for foetal assessment if blood tests suggest an acute infection in pregnancy.
- For immunisation against rubella see p. 199.

 Rubella is a notifiable disease.

TRAVEL HEALTH

The field of travel medicine has grown dramatically in recent years as increasing numbers of people travel to exotic and remote destinations. It is estimated that 600 million people cross international borders annually, and in 2001 a record 58.2 million people travelled abroad from the UK. The knowledge of foreign destinations is not matched by an awareness of the necessary travel precautions, and so the the role of the nurse in primary care in providing comprehensive and up-to-date information to travellers is crucial.

Travel health history
The following may prove a useful aide memoire when obtaining a detailed travel history:

- Date of birth – aids in determining which vaccines are needed, suitable malaria prophylaxis, etc.
- Children's weight – necessary for accurate chemoprophylaxis dosages.
- Family history – important when determining suitable antimalarial prophylaxis or a possible predisposition to thromboembolic disease.
- Pre-existing medical conditions – may preclude certain immunisations or chemoprophylaxis and may require specific health promotion advice.
- Current medication – often highlights existing disease that the individual may not have mentioned presuming that it has no relevance to travel, e.g. it is not unusual for a person whose asthma is well controlled to omit to mention that they are asthmatic. Drug interactions must be considered.
- Previous medical history – this may have implications for chemoprophylaxis, immunisations and individual health advice.
- Previous immunisation history.
- Previous experience of malaria chemoprophylaxis – this will help the practitioner and the traveller to decide on appropriate therapy.
- Contraception – may help to ensure that the traveller is not pregnant at the time of immunisation. The contraceptve pill can be ineffective if combined with doxycycline or if the traveller experiences diarrhoea during the course of their travels.

Continued

Travel health history – *continued*

- Pregnancy – pregnant women not only require special advice on all aspects of their travel, but may often be precluded from being suitably immunised and are limited in their choice of malaria chemoprophylaxis.
- Date of departure – this has implications for planning an immunisation schedule and for determining disease seasonality. Travellers should be encouraged to seek advice about immunisation at least 2 months prior to travel, and if they are regular travellers, to ensure that vaccinations are kept up to date, i.e typhoid every 3 years.
- Duration of stay – the longer the stay in certain areas, the greater the risk factors for certain diseases, e.g. hepatitis A or Japanese encephalitis.
- Location – travellers to remote areas in developing countries may need special immunisation such as rabies. Malaria risk is greater in rural than in urban areas.
- Mode of transport – this has implications for people prone to motion sickness or thromboembolic disease.
- Destinations, including stopovers – yellow fever may not be present in the traveller's ultimate destination, but if stopping in an endemic area immunisation may be required as a condition of entry.
- Planned activities at destination – vaccines such as hepatitis B are not usually advised for short-term travel, but may be recommended if the traveller is to have close contact with the local populace, e.g. aid workers, or those known to indulge in unsafe sex. Malaria prophylaxis is not normally recommended for travel to a country such as South Africa, unless a safari is contemplated.
- Accomodation type – the more basic the accomodation, the greater the risk of exposure to disease caused by biting insects or poor hygiene

For information about individual vaccines see separate headings, and for further information for patients and health professionals, see useful addresses (p. 384).

Advice

Whilst accurate information about immunisation against infectious disease is extremely important, this should also be supported by advice on how to stay healthy whilst abroad.

This advice should include:

- Avoidance of DVT on flights, by wearing flight socks, reducing immobilty as much as is practical, avoiding excess alcohol or sleeping tablets that increase immobility, and remaining adequately hydrated throughout the flight.
- Safe sex, stressing the importance of using condoms that carry the BSI kitemark and the European CE mark, as these have undergone thorough quality checks.

- Sun avoidance advice – cover up exposed skin, avoid midday sun, use sunscreen.
- Food and water – follow local recommendations regarding the safety of drinking water, but, as a rule, avoid ice in drinks, eat fruit that can be peeled and avoid food from street vendors.
- Avoid insect bites by covering exposed skin at dusk, using insect repellent containing DEET, and using impregnated nets where mosquitoes are prevalent.

In many areas it is difficult to source travel health equipment. Selling equipment in the surgery will not only generate practice income, but will enable the health professionals to demonstrate the correct use of the equipment.

Equipment that can be sold includes: • mosquitoe nets and reimpregnation kits • insect repellants • plug-in insecticides • emergency needle and syringe kits • sunscreens • flight socks.

EAR, NOSE AND THROAT

DEAFNESS

Ear wax is the commonest cause of reduced hearing in general practice but it rarely causes deafness.

Diagnosis

History Ask the patient:
- whether the deafness is unilateral or bilateral, and whether the deafness was of sudden onset or gradual onset
- if there are any associated symptoms, such as tinnitus or vertigo, which may suggest a labyrinthine disorder
- whether any drugs have been taken which may affect the acoustic nerve, such as streptomycin and gentamicin.

In the case of children, the parents' account of hearing loss or delayed speech development must be taken seriously.

Examination
- Test the hearing with a whispered voice in each ear in turn.
- Examine to exclude wax, otitis media and a perforated eardrum. (The canal needs to be completely blocked before wax can be held responsible for the hearing loss.)
- Decide whether the problem is conductive or sensorineural using Weber's and Rinne's tuning fork tests.

Weber's test For Weber's test, place the foot of a vibrating tuning fork on the vertex of the patient's skull and ask in which ear the sound is loudest. An asymmetrical Weber's test indicates conductive deafness on the loud side or sensorineural deafness on the quiet side.

Rinne's test In Rinne's test, place the foot of a vibrating tuning fork on the patient's mastoid process. As soon as the sound fades away, hold the tines of the same tuning fork by the external auditory meatus. The normal ear should be able to hear the noise from the tines after the sound from the foot has faded. In Rinne's test, if bone conduction is louder than air conduction, a conductive loss is likely.

Management
Children with hearing loss and glue ear need considering for grommet insertion. For management of occlusive wax by ear syringing, see page 336.

Referral

Unilateral sensorineural hearing loss, even of gradual onset, should be referred urgently once detected in case of acoustic neuroma.

> ⚠ **If sudden hearing loss is sensorineural, and especially if it is unilateral, refer to ENT immediately as there is the possibility of a labyrinthine artery embolism.**

If the principal symptom is bilateral hearing loss and there is no external or middle ear problem to account for it, refer to ENT outpatients. In the elderly this is the commonest scenario and is due to the presbyacusis of old age. It can be helped by a hearing aid, which may be obtained by referral to the ENT outpatient department, or by direct referral to a hearing aid department.

Administration
Referral to a social worker for the deaf may be helpful, if this has not been done by the hospital.

THE DISCHARGING EAR

The commonest cause of discharging ear in general practice is otitis externa. It is usually unilateral.

Diagnosis
History Ask about: • any tendency to excessive ear wax • earache • the likelihood of a foreign body in the ear • bleeding and deafness associated with the discharge.

Examination Examine the ear, looking for: • wax • a foreign body • otitis externa • otitis media • a furuncle • perforated eardrum.

Investigations Take a swab of the discharge and send it to bacteriology.

Management
Wax If wax is discharging from the ear it should not need treating. If it is irritating the patient, advise sodium bicarbonate eardrops t.d.s. for 4–5 days, then syringe the ear if the problem has not resolved (see p. 336).

Foreign body Remove any foreign body, if accessible; refer if not.

Otitis externa See page 219.

Otitis media See page 218.

Perforated eardrum Perforations of the eardrum usually heal spontaneously within 4–6 weeks. The perforated eardrum may require referral to ENT if healing has not occurred within 6 weeks. If the perforation is near the margin of the eardrum, as opposed to the centre, consider an earlier referral; cholesteatoma can present as a chronic discharging ear with a marginal perforation.

EARACHE

Earache can be very painful and makes children miserable. Parents of small children soon learn the importance of keeping a stock of paediatric paracetamol in the house.

Diagnosis

History Ask about:
- Any symptoms of an upper respiratory tract infection. Patients with colds who develop earache will usually have either otitis media or eustachian tube dysfunction.
- Other causes include:
  - otitis externa
  - trauma to the canal
  - foreign body
  - perforation of the drum as a result of otitis media (accompanied by the relief of pain).
- Unusual causes to consider are:
  - shingles
  - temporomandibular joint dysfunction
  - mastoiditis
  - toothache.

Examination If the eardrum is red, bulging or dull, middle ear infection is suspected. If the eardrum is normal, eustachian tube dysfunction is likely, i.e. increased pressure in the middle ear due to a blocked eustachian tube.

Look also for: • a boil in the canal • the vesicular rash of shingles • inflammation behind the earlobe, suggesting mastoiditis.

Investigations Take a swab of any discharge from the ear and send it to bacteriology.

Management

Otitis media It is reasonable to treat cases of acute otitis media with regular analgesia such as paracetamol. Recent evidence suggests that acute otitis media in children can be effectively managed with analgesia alone. Antibiotics such as amoxycillin 125 mg t.d.s. under 3 years of age, 250 mg t.d.s. over 3 years, may be given

Eustachian tube dysfunction For eustachian tube dysfunction advise regular analgesia and warm drinks. (The action of swallowing helps.) The role of decongestants is more controversial.

Otitis externa For otitis externa prescribe an antibiotic eardrop, such as gentamicin HC eardrops, with or without an oral antibiotic, such as amoxycillin. If there has been no response in 1 week, try an alternative eardrop, e.g. Otosporin or Locorten, with or without oral erythromycin. Refer for aural toilet if there is no response.

Wax Ear wax can be painful, but usually responds to the use of olive oil eardrops for 1–2 weeks. Syringing may be necessary if the wax persists (see p. 336).

Boil A boil in the ear canal requires analgesics. Antibiotics or incision and drainage may be necessary if the pain is severe.

Shingles See page 188.

 If mastoiditis is suspected, refer the patient to ENT urgently.

Temporomandibular joint dysfunction This also requires analgesics. Reassure the patient that the condition is self-limiting.

Toothache This is best dealt with by prescribing analgesics and advising patients to contact their dentist. For dental abscesses also prescribe penicillin V and metronidazole (see p. 226).

Perforated eardrum See page 217.

TINNITUS

Tinnitus is a ringing, buzzing, hissing or pulsating in the ears.

Diagnosis

History Ask about associated symptoms, e.g.: • hearing loss • dizziness • earache.

Examination
• Check the ears for otitis media, otitis externa and wax.
• Check BP.

Investigations FBC to exclude anaemia.

Management

- Patients with tinnitus often present for the first time with fear of a sinister underlying disease, such as a brain tumour or high blood pressure. Reassure the patient if appropriate.
- The majority of cases resolve. Distraction techniques, such as increasing background noise, are often useful.
- Treat wax or otitis if present.
- If there is no response and the patient is still suffering, referral to ENT outpatients is indicated.
- 'Maskers' are available through ENT outpatients.
- Suggest the British Tinnitus Association for educational support (see p. 384).

> In Ménière's disease and other longstanding causes of tinnitus, patients should be told that drug treatment is ineffective and that, while the ringing will not go away, they will gradually become less aware of it.

HAY FEVER

In some areas hay fever is the commonest condition presenting to GPs in May and June.

Diagnosis

History Hay fever is characterised by the variable combination of: • seasonal rhinitis • conjunctivitis • occasionally, sore throat and wheeze.

Examination Examination is usually unnecessary, but it may be necessary to exclude infective conjunctivitis. (Swab if in doubt.)

Management

Advise the patient to avoid situations in which exposure to pollen will be highest – being outside in the evening, driving with car windows open, sleeping with bedroom window open.

- Prescribe an oral antihistamine, e.g. Desloratadine 5 mg o.d. or Cetirizine 10 mg o.d. Some preparations are available OTC.
- Steroid nasal sprays are useful for the rhinitis of hay fever, e.g. beclomethasone, two sprays b.d. per nostril.
- Mast cell stabilisers, e.g. sodium cromoglycate eyedrops, two drops q.d.s., help relieve allergic conjunctivitis.
- A bronchodilator inhaler, e.g. salbutamol, may be needed for wheezing.

A stepwise approach to prescribing will reduce costs, but a combination of the four types of treatment will often be necessary.

EPISTAXIS

Patients with nosebleeds present in general practice both acutely, with bleeding, and afterwards, for the prevention of recurrence.

Diagnosis

History Ask how much blood has been lost, which nostril the blood comes from and whether the patient has any disorder of blood clotting.

Examination Measure BP. Look up the nose to try to identify a bleeding point. Little's area, on the nasal septum just inside the nostril, often contains some large, delicate blood vessels.

Management

Nosebleeds are very common in young children and are often recurrent. No specific preventive treatment is necessary, as the tendency often remits spontaneously.

To stop acute bleeding
- Advise the patient or parent to squeeze the nose just below the bony part of the nasal bridge. The pressure needs applying continuously for 15 minutes, and it is best if this is timed with a watch. This stops most bleeds.
- If the bleeding does not stop within 15 minutes of continuous pressure, admit the patient. Alternatively, pack the nose with an adrenaline-soaked wick by pushing it gently towards the *back* of the nasal cavity with McGill forceps. A nasal balloon catheter may be used instead. Admit the patient if this does not control the bleeding.

To prevent further bleeding
- The recurrent bleeding nose is probably best cauterised. If a bleeding point can be identified in Little's area the blood vessel can be touched with the tip of a silver nitrate stick.
- Consider referral for nasal cautery if the bleeding point cannot be identified.

BLOCKED NOSE

Nasal obstruction can be either bilateral or unilateral, although distinguishing between the two is of little diagnostic use in general practice, except when a foreign body in the nose is suspected. A more useful distinction is between acute blockage (of a few days) and chronic blockage (of, say, more than 3 weeks).

ACUTE BLOCKAGE

Diagnosis

History Ask about: • symptoms of upper respiratory tract infection (URTI) • the likelihood of a foreign body • a blood clot following a nosebleed.
  Consider also trauma (septal haematoma) and hay fever.

Examination Using the largest auroscope, look up each nostril for:
• a foreign body, if suspected
• a septal haematoma, if there is a history of trauma
• the hyperaemia of Little's area associated with nosebleeds (see p. 221).

Management

If symptoms warrant treatment in an URTI, advise normal saline nose drops. Failing this, xylometazoline nose drops will help if used for a short while.

Hay fever See page 220.

Sinusitis The blocked nose of acute sinusitis is associated with yellow, green or blood-streaked nasal discharge and facial tenderness. Treat with amoxycillin or doxycycline. For chronic sinusitis, treat initially with steroid sprays or decongestants, e.g. beclomethasone two sprays b.d. per nostril. Otherwise, refer for sinus X-rays or CT and antral lavage if indicated.

CHRONIC BLOCKAGE

Diagnosis

History Ask about:
• Nasal speech and the tendency to nasal discharge during URTIs. This may suggest:
  – adenoid hyperplasia
  – nasal polyps
  – septal mucosal hyperplasia.
• Sleep apnoea syndrome in adults, in which the sleep is interrupted by respiratory tract blockage at night, making daytime sleepiness a problem. This has been associated with chronic nasal blockage.
• Glue ear (in children) and snoring, which can also result from chronic nasal obstruction.

Examination Examination is often normal in general practice.

Management

Nasal steroid sprays, e.g. beclomethasone, may provide partial relief, as will treatment of acute infective exacerbations with antibiotics.

Referral Referral for e.g. adenoidectomy should be considered for nasal speech, recurrent infections, sleep apnoea or glue ear in children, and for e.g. submucous resection or polypectomy, if appropriate, on failure of medical treatment in adults.

SORE THROAT

Acute viral or streptococcal sore throats are a very common feature of general practice. Glandular fever, quinsy and the sore throat of postnasal drip in sinusitis are less common.

Diagnosis

History Ask about:
- The duration of the symptoms: most acute viral and streptococcal sore throats get better spontaneously within 5–7 days.
- Symptoms of systemic illness: fever, sweating, myalgia and fatigue all suggest a more severe infection.
- The patient's expectations: some patients expect a prescription for antibiotics; others want reassurance or a medical certificate.

Examination
- Examine the throat with a good light.
- Look for the presence of pus on the tonsils, suggesting tonsillitis, and for the creamy white film of glandular fever.
- Palpate the cervical lymph nodes.

Investigations Investigations are usually unnecessary and unhelpful in the majority of cases of sore throat. Throat swabs take at least 3 days to give a result, by which time most patients are better.

Blood-testing for glandular fever becomes more sensitive after the first 3 weeks, so repeat the test if a first early test is negative and the patient is no better 1–2 weeks later.

Management

Viral infections Viral throat infections are best treated with analgesics. Antiseptic or analgesic mouthwashes may also help.

Bacterial infections In streptococcal throat infections the duration of the illness can probably be shortened by 24 hours with the use of penicillin.

(Unfortunately there is no quick way of distinguishing between viral and bacterial throat infections. The use of antibiotics is therefore difficult to justify.) If the patient is toxic, prescribe an antibiotic that is effective against streptococci, e.g. penicillin V, or erythromycin, 250 mg q.d.s. for 5 days.

Quinsy Painful, marked swelling of a single tonsil suggests a quinsy, especially if a collection of pus can be seen to point from within the tonsil. Refer the patient to ENT casualty for incision and drainage.

Glandular fever This should be considered if there is a film over the tonsils. Cervical lymphadenopathy is usually marked. Petechiae on the palate and hepatosplenomegaly may also be present. Avoid amoxycillin, as the development of a rash is common. There is no specific treatment for the infection, but analgesics are often useful in reducing the soreness in the throat.

Chronic sore throat Consider physical causes of irritation of the throat, such as snoring, dust inhalation, gastro-oesophageal reflux.

Recurrent sore throat Reinfection within families is a cause of recurrent throat infection, particularly with *Streptococcus pyogenes*. Send a throat swab and treat the family with penicillin or erythromycin if positive.

 If a patient on carbimazole develops a sore throat, consider neutropenia. Check an FBC urgently.

Mouth ulcers See page 226.

CERVICAL LYMPHADENOPATHY

The isolated, enlarged lymph node in the neck is usually an associated finding with URTIs. Enlarged lymph nodes occasionally present alone, either with tenderness or without.

Diagnosis

History Ask about symptoms relating to the following possible diagnoses:
• sore throat • earache • runny nose • scalp laceration • scalp infection
• pyrexial illness.

Examination Examine the ears, nose and throat, and the scalp if necessary. Consider looking for other glands in the axillae and groins (and liver and spleen for thoroughness).

Management

- Often the cause is a non-specific viral illness and the gland returns to its normal state after a few weeks.
- Treat any underlying infection, as appropriate.
- If no infection can be found it is reasonable to wait and see for 4–6 weeks in the absence of other symptoms.
- If the gland remains enlarged, an FBC with differential white count and a Paul–Bunnell test will reveal any haematological malignancies and glandular fever. If the blood tests are negative, refer the patient to the ENT outpatient department for a biopsy to exclude tuberculosis or malignancy.

HOARSENESS

Hoarseness and loss of voice commonly present in general practice as acute problems in association with URTIs. Acute viral laryngitis is the usual cause, for which the treatment is symptomatic: analgesia for the sore throat and resting the voice.

Diagnosis

If the problem lasts more than a few weeks, consider the following diagnoses: • overuse of the voice (e.g. singing) • snoring • oropharyngeal thrush (e.g. from steroid inhalers) • hypothyroidism • carcinoma of the larynx or lung (recurrent laryngeal nerve palsy) • vocal cord disease.

Investigations Baseline tests include: • FBC • TFTs • CXR.

Management

- Manage any of the specific diseases above, if detected.
- Rest the voice if it is being overused.
- If inhalers cause thrush, advise the patient to rinse the mouth out after use. Nystatin oral suspension or amphotericin lozenges will help.
- Refer the patient to ENT if in doubt.

> ⚠️ **All patients with unexplained hoarseness for more than 3 weeks need referral to ENT to exclude carcinoma of the larynx.**

GUM DISEASE

DENTAL ABSCESS

A dental abscess produces a painful tender swelling of the cheek adjacent to an infected tooth root. Often the carious tooth can be identified. It is worth excluding a parotid gland swelling by making sure the angle of the jaw is palpable.

Management
Prescribe analgesia, e.g. co-proxamol, two tablets 4-hourly, and antibiotics, such as penicillin V 500 mg 6-hourly and metronidazole 800 mg 8-hourly.
Refer patients to their dentist.

GINGIVITIS

Gingivitis is inflammation of the gums, making them fragile and prone to bleeding on brushing. It occurs in the presence of dental caries, although not exclusively.

Management
Advise patients on general dental hygiene and suggest they see a dental hygienist. Chlorhexidine oral rinse 0.2% is useful in some cases.

MOUTH ULCERS

Painful acute ulceration is nearly always benign, but consider carcinoma of the oral cavity for ulcers that do not resolve over 6 weeks.

Management
- Mouth ulcers are usually aphthous, but can occasionally be viral. Most respond to symptomatic treatment with an analgesic oral gel.
- Prescribe nystatin oral suspension 1 ml q.d.s. if thrush is likely.
- Adcortyl in Orabase applied to the ulcers often speeds up the healing.
- Benzydamine spray is useful for ulcers of the tongue.

SNORING

Snoring affects everyone some of the time, and some people most of the time! Most requests for medical help come from partners whose sleep is affected by the patient's snoring.
In most cases of snoring the cause is unknown, or due to obesity.

History Ask about:
- weight
- neck size
- alcohol intake
- nasal obstruction
- day-time somnolence.

Examination Look for:
- nasal polyps
- septal deviation
- enlarged tonsils
- enlarged uvula.

Management

Advise weight loss if the BMI is greater than 26 kg/m² or if the collar size is greater than 17 inches.

Advise alcohol moderation in drinkers.

For nasal obstruction advise the use of AirFlow nasal plasters, or Nozovent. Both these are devices for holding the nostrils open at night, and are available from most pharmacies.

Referral

Refer to the ENT department patients with severe snoring, nasal polyps, tonsilar or uvular hypertrophy, deviated nasal septum or suspicious lesions in the head or neck.

Refer to a sleep clinic or local chest physician if the patient complains of daytime somnolence. Sleep apnoea can be a complication of snoring, especially in patients with a collar size greater than 17 inches. This condition is treatable with continuous positive pressure ventilation via a nasal mask at night.

OPHTHALMOLOGY

THE DISCHARGING EYE

Eyes water as a result of either excessive tear production or inadequate tear drainage.

Excessive tear production

Common causes • Wind • dust • ingrowing eyelash • corneal or tarsal foreign body • hay fever.

Impaired tear drainage

Common causes • URTI • ectropion • entropion • blocked tear duct.

Diagnosis

History Ask about symptoms of URTI, allergy and possible trauma.

Examination
- Examine the cornea for foreign bodies.
- Inspect the eyelids for:
  - ectropion
  - entropion
  - ingrowing eyelash
  - the presence of an eyelash in the tear duct
  - signs of conjunctivitis.
- Evert the eyelid if the history suggests a foreign body in the eye.

Management

For a chronically sticky eye in a baby, show the parents how to massage the lacrimal duct with gentle pressure from the index finger over the medial palpebral fold twice daily. Also, use antibiotic eyedrops if the eye is red. Regular swabbing with moistened cotton wool helps. Refer for duct probing under anaesthetic if there has been no improvement by 6 months of age.

Eyelashes in the tear duct can be easily removed with fine forceps.

Refer the patient with an ectropion, entropion or ingrowing eyelash for corrective surgery. Avoid drops or ointment unless obvious conjunctivitis is present.

THE DRY EYE

Dry eye is a symptom that has many causes. The patient may mean gritty, sore, irritating or even painful eye (see p. 236).

Diagnosis

History Ask about known conditions that may cause the eyes to be dry. The commonest are idiopathic and old age.

Conjunctivitis commonly causes the eye to feel dry. The symptoms also include itching, a sticky discharge and a bloodshot appearance.

Other rare causes are: • Sjögren's syndrome (rheumatoid arthritis) • sarcoidosis • *Chlamydia trachomatis* infection • exposure keratitis • Stevens–Johnson syndrome • pemphigoid.

Examination Look for signs of infection, ectropion and entropion.

Investigations A conjunctival swab may be indicated in conjunctivitis. Schirmer's test, in which a strip of special blotting paper is hung from the lower lid margin, may give an idea of the degree of dryness, but in practice is of little help in the management of the dry eye.

Management

- Give antibiotic eyedrops for suspected conjunctivitis.
- Hypromellose eyedrops p.r.n. are often the most useful treatment for the chronically dry eye.
- Manage any underlying disease as appropriate.
- Refer for eye surgery in cases of ectropion and entropion.

EYELID PROBLEMS

STYE

Styes are very common. They are infected eyelash roots and produce a red, painful swelling at the lid margin.

Management

Advise regular hot steaming. Once the stye is pointing, the affected lash can be pulled out, discharging the pus and relieving the pain. Antibiotic eyedrops, e.g. chloramphenicol, can be prescribed.

MEIBOMIAN CYST (CHALAZION)

Chalazions are less common than styes and produce a red, uncomfortable swelling in the middle of the eyelid.

Management

For the acute infection advise regular hot steaming and antibiotic eyedrops, e.g. chloramphenicol. The cyst usually bursts through the conjunctiva.

If the problem is recurrent or if the cyst remains, consider referral to an ophthamologist for incision and curettage.

BLEPHARITIS

Blepharitis is chronic inflammation of the lid margins. It gives the eyes a sore, tired appearance, with red lid margins.

Management
- Advise the patient to avoid rubbing the eyes and pay attention to cleaning the lid margins carefully with warm water.
- Baby lotion wiped over the lid margins with cotton wool often helps, as does an antibiotic eye ointment.
- Treat any associated seborrhoeic dermatitis.

SQUINT

A squint is a misalignment of the visual axes of the two eyes. It is normal in very new babies, until they are old enough to focus on near objects.

Diagnosis

History
- When does the child have the squint (e.g. when tired)?
- Ask if there have been any developmental problems.

Examination Attempt to confirm the squint, as prominent epicanthic folds often give the false impression of a squint.

The corneal light reflex With the child looking at the light from a pen torch from a distance of about half a metre, the reflection of the light is symmetrical in the non-squinting child.

The cover test Get the child to look at a small toy. Cover one eye while observing the other eye. If the uncovered eye moves to take up fixation on the toy, he or she probably has a squint.

The red reflex In babies check for the rare conditions retinoblastoma, retinitis pigmentosa and cataract using the red reflex. Observe the eyes through the ophthalmoscope from a distance of 20 cm. The normal eye has a uniformly red reflection in the middle of the pupil. Any abnormality of this reflex is suspicious.

Management

 If there is an abnormal red reflex, refer immediately.

- If the squint is confirmed, routine referral to the ophthalmology outpatient department is indicated.
- If a squint is not confirmed, refer if the history is convincing. The latent squint may appear only when the child is tired. Otherwise reassure the parents and offer to review the patient in 6 months.
- Reassure the parents that most squints can be corrected without surgery, e.g. by the use of patching or spectacles.

THE ACUTE RED EYE

There are many causes of red eye, even in general practice. The lists below give the principal distinguishing features.

- **Most red eyes in general practice are not painful.**
- **The acute, painful, red eye usually needs urgent referral to ophthalmology.**
- **The very painful, red eye should be referred immediately.**

Diagnosis

History
- Assess the level of pain.
- Ask about visual acuity. (Test if in doubt.)
- Is there any discharge?
- Is there any photophobia?
- Could there be a risk of a foreign body in the eye?

Differential diagnosis

Causes of the painless red eye
- Conjunctivitis.
- Subconjunctival haemorrhage.

Causes of the painful red eye
- Corneal abrasion.
- Herpes zoster infection.
- Arc eye/snow blindness.
- Corneal foreign body.
- Episcleritis and scleritis.
- Acute glaucoma.
- Acute iritis.
- Acute keratitis.

CONJUNCTIVITIS

Conjunctivitis is the most common eye condition seen by GPs. It is usually seen in the context of an upper respiratory tract infection or hay fever.

Diagnosis

History Irritation, grittiness, dryness, itching, stinging or soreness are common complaints in conjunctivitis. In most straightforward cases this is followed by the bloodshot eye, and discharging green/yellow sticky pus which glues the eyelids together overnight.

Any combination of the above symptoms may occur.

 If the eye is painful, consider an alternative diagnosis.

Examination Look for: • vasodilation of the conjunctiva • cobblestone oedema of the conjunctiva under the eyelids • purulent discharge.

Differential diagnosis • See: the acute red eye (p. 233) • the dry eye (p. 230) • the painful eye (p. 236) • the discharging eye (p. 230).

Management
- In obvious or suspected cases it is reasonable to start treatment with chloramphenicol eye ointment t.d.s. or drops q.d.s. for a few days.
- If there is no response, a swab of the discharge can be sent for microscopy, culture and sensitivities. At the same time, the treatment can be changed to fusidic acid eyedrops b.d. for a further week.
- In hay fever, the conjunctivitis is likely to be allergic, and treatment with antihistamine tablets, e.g. desloratadine 5 mg o.d., or eyedrops, e.g. sodium cromoglycate q.d.s., should be tried initially.
- If there is no response, consider referral.

Infective conjunctivitis is contagious and patients should be advised not to share towels or flannels. It is not necessary to avoid school once treatment has been started.

SUBCONJUNCTIVAL HAEMORRHAGE

- Common.
- Completely painless.
- Normal acuity.
- No discharge or photophobia.
- No trauma.
- Usually only a part of the cornea is densely red.
- The pupil is normal.

Management

No treatment is usually required as spontaneous resolution occurs.

CORNEAL ABRASION

- Frequent.
- Mild to moderate pain.
- Acuity sometimes slightly reduced.
- Watering eye; no discharge.
- Little or no photophobia.
- Usually a history of mild trauma.
- Fluorescein stain is taken up by exposed keratin.

Management

Apply amethocaine drops, chloramphenicol ointment and an eyepad initially. Thereafter use antibiotic ointment t.d.s.

Review after 24 hours to check for healing.

HERPES ZOSTER INFECTION

- Not uncommon.
- Periorbital vesicular rash.
- Watering eye.
- Soreness.

Management

Refer urgently, to exclude a dendritic ulcer. Treat with oral aciclovir or valaciclovir.

ARC EYE/SNOW BLINDNESS

- Uncommon in general practice.
- Moderate to severe pain.
- Slightly decreased acuity.
- Watering eye.
- Some photophobia.
- History of exposure to welding arc or snow.

Management

Anaesthetic eyedrops and an eyepad are usually sufficient, as spontaneous resolution occurs rapidly.

CORNEAL FOREIGN BODY

- Uncommon in general practice.
- Moderate pain.
- Slightly decreased acuity.
- Watering eye.
- Little or no photophobia.
- A history of something going into the eye.
- A foreign body is usually visible on the surface of the cornea or under the eyelids. (These may need everting.)

Management

Apply amethocaine drops. Remove the foreign body with a needlepoint under magnification. Consider the possibility of an intraocular foreign body.

Prescribe chloramphenicol ointment t.d.s. and apply a pad for 4 hours. Check for the presence of a rust ring after 24 hours.

Alternatively, the patient may be encouraged to attend the local eye casualty department.

THE PAINFUL EYE

A useful distinction to make in general practice is between the red painful eye and the normal-looking painful eye.

THE RED PAINFUL EYE

See page 233.

THE NORMAL-LOOKING PAINFUL EYE

Possible causes of the normal looking painful eye:

- Commonly:
  - long-sightedness
  - migraine
  - sinusitis
  - stress headache.
- Rarely:
  - dental pain
  - retrobulbar neuritis
  - temporal arteritis
  - temporomandibular joint dysfunction.

SUDDEN VISUAL LOSS

⚠ Sudden loss of vision is an ophthalmological emergency and requires immediate referral to hospital.

Causes
- Retinal artery embolus.
- Retinal vein thrombosis.
- Retinal detachment.
- Acute angle closure glaucoma.
- Giant cell arteritis.
- Retrobulbar neuritis.

Immediate management
Most of these conditions can be adequately dealt with by arranging immediate transfer of the patient to the eye emergency department.

If there is likely to be any delay, there are two conditions for which treatment started at home or in the surgery can save sight: • giant cell (temporal) arteritis • acute angle closure glaucoma.

GIANT CELL (TEMPORAL) ARTERITIS

Diagnosis

History The patient is elderly and complains of a temporal headache and tenderness, accompanied by blurring or loss of vision in one eye.

Examination Examination reveals a tender, hardened temporal artery and perhaps a mild fever. The eye looks normal.

Management

In the presence of such typical features take blood for ESR and give prednisolone 80 mg p.o. Arrange for the patient to go to hospital as soon as possible. A temporal artery biopsy can then be arranged to try and help confirm the diagnosis. See also p. 248.

ACUTE ANGLE CLOSURE GLAUCOMA

Diagnosis

History The patient has a severely painful red eye, may be vomiting, and complains of having seen haloes around lights.

Examination Examination reveals a cloudy cornea and a dilated pupil compared with the good eye.

Management

Instillation of 4% pilocarpine drops every minute for 5 minutes, then every 5 minutes will reduce the intraocular pressure. If available, an injection of 500 mg of acetazolamide i.v. will also help. Alternatively, a 250 mg acetazolamide tablet can be given if the patient is not vomiting. Arrange for the patient to go to hospital as soon as possible.

OTHER CAUSES

Cerebrovascular accident

The sudden onset of a homonymous hemianopia associated with a stroke is not unusual but can occasionally be the only neurological consequence of a posterior cerebral artery infarct. Referral is indicated for complete neurological assessment and rehabilitation.

Migraine

The visual changes accompanying a migraine attack are usually described as flashing lights, blurred vision or spots or zigzags, rather than loss of vision. If visual loss is reported as a presenting complaint for the first time, even in the presence of a migrainous headache, it is probably wise to discuss the case with the duty ophthalmologist.

PROGRESSIVE VISUAL LOSS

Children and young adults with progressive visual loss should be referred to an ophthalmologist. The causes in this group include: • refractive error • amblyopia of disuse • diabetic retinopathy • inherited retinal degeneration (e.g. retinitis pigmentosa) • posterior uveitis • pituitary tumour.

Adults with gradual blurring of the vision can be encouraged to see an optician first. They are most likely to need only spectacles.

The commonest causes of progressive visual loss in the elderly

- Refractive error.
- Cataract.
- Senile macular degeneration.
- Chronic open-angle glaucoma.
- Hypertensive retinopathy.

Diagnosis

History Ask about:

- pre-existing diseases that are known to affect the sight, e.g. diabetes, hypertension, thyroid disorder
- the extent to which the loss of vision affects the patient, e.g. driving, reading, general mobility
- the speed of onset of the visual loss.

Examination

- Measure the visual acuity (VA) with a Snellen chart and record the results. A VA of 6/36 means the patient can read at 6 m what the average person can read at 36 m, i.e. only the bigger letters. Normal vision is a VA of 6/6.
- Check BP.
- Screen for diabetes.
- Assess the visual fields with confrontation testing, to exclude the peripheral visual field loss of chronic open-angle glaucoma.
- Examine for cataract (see p. 240).

Management

Referral to an ophthalmologist is indicated in most cases of visual loss. The timing of the referral depends on a number of factors, including the suspected cause and the patient's need to try and recover some of the lost vision (see cataract, below).

Registration of a patient as partially sighted or blind is the statutory duty of the consultant ophthalmologist, not the GP.

Advice Benefits and aids for the partially sighted are many. Refer the patient to the social worker for the blind unless this has already been done.

Inform the patient of the existence of the Royal National Institute for the Blind (see p. 387) and any local clubs for the blind and partially sighted.

CATARACT

Cataract, or lens opacity, affects approximately 25% of the population in the 65–75-year age range.

Diagnosis

History Ask about progressive decrease in VA, and glare.

Examination Look at the eye through an ophthalmoscope from a distance of 20 cm. The normal homogeneous red reflex is obscured by dark lines across the pupil. Fundoscopy is often difficult due to the obstructed view.

Differential diagnosis See progressive visual loss (p. 239).

Management

The mainstay of treatment for cataract is surgical, but the timing of the referral will depend on a number of factors. As soon as the VA has deteriorated enough to affect the patient's usual daily routine, he or she should be referred for a surgical opinion. Allowances should be made for long waiting lists.

In the meantime, advise patients not to drive if they fail to meet the standards required by the Driver and Vehicle Licensing Agency, i.e. to be able to read a number plate at 67 ft (20 m) with either eye.

CHRONIC GLAUCOMA

Chronic open-angle glaucoma is usually suspected by finding a raised intraocular pressure, cupping of the optic discs or peripheral visual field loss on charting. These changes are usually detected by the optician on routine eye testing.

Referral to the ophthalmology outpatient department is indicated.

Confirmed cases are followed up in outpatients. Treatment usually consists of eyedrops to either reduce intraocular pressure or facilitate anterior chamber drainage. Occasionally, surgery is indicated (iridocentesis).

Issues for the GP include:

- Family members are at increased risk of chronic glaucoma.
- Repeat prescribing of eyedrops.

- Beta blocker eyedrops can have systemic effects in e.g. asthma and heart failure.
- Management of progressive visual loss (see p. 239).

FLOATERS

Floaters are small, black spots, seen by the patient to be floating in front of the eyes. They are very common and patients need reassuring that there is likely to be nothing wrong with their eyes.

The fortification spectra of migraine may be described as black spots, but these are usually followed by the headache and are temporary.

Management
Nothing need usually be done, other than to reassure the patient that the condition is benign and usually self-limiting.

> ⚠ **If the floaters are described as large, dark blobs which appear suddenly and are associated with flashing lights, the cause may be retinal detachment and the patient should be referred immediately.**

Occasionally the patient may have a cataract (see p. 240).

RHEUMATOLOGY AND ORTHOPAEDICS

JOINT PAIN

Many patients present with multiple aches and pains and some of these may be described as joint pains.

Diagnosis

History Ask about:
- The duration of symptoms: a short-term illness requires a diagnosis. In long-term problems, first find out what the patient wants: symptom relief or reassurance.
- Associated features such as viral illness, depression or fatigue.
- Generalised or localised symptoms.
- Diurnal symptoms.
- Joint stiffness.

Examination Look at:
- the affected area for inflammation, deformity or restricted movement
- nearby structures, such as the neck in shoulder pain
- whether it is a joint problem, periarticular or muscular
- tender spots, as in tennis elbow and fibrositis
- other areas as suggested by the history.

Causes of joint pain

It is worth having a checklist of causes of joint pain in mind when seeing these patients. The commonest are given first:

- unaccustomed use
- repeated overuse
- viral illness
- osteoarthritis (see p. 247).
- non-articular rheumatic pain, e.g. tennis elbow (see p. 254)
- gout (see p. 245)
- polymyalgia rheumatica (see p. 248)
- rheumatoid arthritis (see p. 250)
- other connective tissue disorders
- malignancy and myeloma.

Investigations If the diagnosis remains unclear having taken a careful history and examined the relevant parts, bloods can be requested for FBC, ESR or CRP, rheumatoid factor and serum uric acid. See the patient after 2 weeks. Insignificant causes will produce normal results (except, perhaps, for a slightly raised ESR in viral illnesses).

Persistent abnormality prompts management as in the relevant sections listed in the box on page 244, or referral for further diagnostic tests.

GOUT

Gout presents most commonly in middle-aged men. It may affect any joint, but is usually seen in the big toe, ankle or knee.

Diagnosis

History Ask about the spontaneous onset of severe pain in one joint, exacerbated by movement.

Examination Look for:
- inflammation of the joint (red, hot and swollen)
- gouty nodules around ears, bursae or tendons, which suggest chronic gout.

Investigations

Serum uric acid This is usually raised in gout, but is non-specific.

Creatinine and electrolytes In chronic gout it is necessary to exclude kidney damage with a serum creatinine and electrolytes.

Lipids Check for hyperlipidaemia, which often coexists.

Joint aspiration The diagnosis of gout is usually obvious after the history and examination. If in doubt, aspirate fluid from the joint. Uric acid crystals in the synovial fluid are diagnostic.

Management

Advice Give general advice about reducing the risk of gout:
- Reduce alcohol intake
- Avoid being overweight.

Prescribing A therapeutic trial of a strong NSAID (see below) may help to exclude other diseases, as the acute attack of gout should subside within a few days.
   Stop any thiazide diuretics.

- For the acute attack, prescribe indomethacin 50 mg t.d.s. or naproxen 500 mg b.d.
- If the patient has a contraindication to NSAIDs, use colchicine 0.5–1 mg q.d.s.
- For recurrent attacks prescribe allopurinol 100 mg daily. This can be increased, up to 600 mg daily, if attacks recur. Do not start allopurinol until after an attack has subsided.

NECK PAIN

Neck pain is commonly a mild, self-limiting nuisance due possibly to muscle tension.

Diagnosis

History
- Ask about the duration of the symptoms. A short history of neck pain, usually on one side of the neck more than the other and with a twisting of the neck, suggests acute torticollis. This sort of acute pain, but without the twisting, is common in whiplash injuries.
- Ask about chronic pain and stiffness in the neck. These symptoms may be due to degeneration in the cervical intervertebral discs, suggestive of cervical spondylosis. Early morning stiffness may be a feature of osteoarthritis of the cervical spine. Severe neck pain, usually accompanied by occipital headache, suggests meningism, especially in someone not accustomed to neck pain.
- Exclude radiculopathy and myelopathy by asking the patient about symptoms of pain or weakness in the arms or legs.

Examination Look for:
- Tenderness in the neck muscles. If the head is held to one side and the patient cannot straighten the head, think of acute torticollis.
- A reduced range of movement of the cervical spine, which suggests cervical spondylosis or arthritis.
- Weakness and wasting in the arms or legs, which suggest a radiculopathy or myelopathy, not uncommon in cervical spondylosis. Examine for this if there are suggestive symptoms.

Investigations If the diagnosis is in doubt or if the patient is particularly requesting it, an X-ray of the cervical spine is useful. Cervical spondylosis and arthritis usually show up after 6 months of disease.

Management
- Physiotherapy helps to improve the range of pain-free movement in both acute and chronic cases of neck pain.
- A collar often helps by temporarily resting the neck.
- Prescribe NSAIDs or simple analgesics for pain.
- Diazepam tablets 2–5 mg t.d.s. help relieve the muscle spasm of acute torticollis.
- Refer all cases with neurological complications.

OSTEOARTHRITIS

Osteoarthritis is the most common joint disease seen in general practice, its incidence increasing with age. It is a progressive, debilitating disease, mainly affecting the weight-bearing joints and hands.

Diagnosis

History Ask about pain and early morning stiffness, usually in a knee, hip or ankle. Symptoms will have been present for some months and may have been exacerbated by recent injury or overuse.

Examination
- Look for a reduced range of movement or pain on movement of the affected joint or joints.
- Crepitus may be felt by laying a hand on the joint while moving it.
- The soft-tissue swelling of osteoarthritis produces a 'fattened' joint and fluid effusions are often absent.
- The patient may have a limp, use a stick or have difficulty getting on to the examination couch.

Investigation
- X-rays are unhelpful in the early stages of the disease, although 6 months of osteoarthritis will usually show characteristic X-ray changes.
- Blood tests exclude other causes of arthritis (see rheumatoid arthritis, p. 250).

Management

Advice
- Aim for ideal weight.
- Encorage mobility/activity.
- Social services will advise the patient about allowances and benefits and a disabled parking permit.
- Educational leaflets and support groups are a useful source of information for patients.
- Be on the lookout for depression and carer stress.

Treatment
- For the relief of pain, start with simple paracetamol and increase if necessary to co-proxamol or co-dydramol.
- Stiffness can be relieved by NSAIDs. A big evening dose is useful in early morning stiffness, e.g. ibuprofen S/R 800 mg, two tablets nocte.
- Beware of gastric irritation in the elderly. Prescribe an H_2 blocker if necessary.
- Consider a Cox II inhibitor, e.g. rofecoxib 12.5–25 mg o.d. for patients at high risk of developing serious gastrointestinal side-effects (see BNF).

- Consider glucosamine as an alternative for pain releif (only available OTC).
- Physiotherapy is useful for maintaining joint mobility.
- Consider intra-articular injection of corticosteroid if only one or two joints are affected (e.g. for knee joint, methylprednisolone 40 mg).
- Walking aids such as sticks and frames can be obtained by referral to the local occupational therapy or physiotherapy department or from the day hospital.
- Occupational therapy can also help with activities of daily living and modification of the home.

Referral Consider referral for joint replacements. The timing of referral depends on the effect of the disease on the patient's life in terms of immobility and pain. Generally, the patient who is being woken at night despite full doses of anti-inflammatories and non-addictive analgesics should be on the waiting list for surgery.

POLYMYALGIA RHEUMATICA AND GIANT CELL ARTERITIS

Polymyalgia rheumatica is a common condition in Caucasians, mainly affecting women over 55. It coexists with giant cell arteritis in about 30% of cases (see p. 238).

Diagnosis

History

Polymyalgia rheumatica Ask about pain and stiffness around the shoulders or, occasionally, the hips, which is worse in the mornings.

Giant cell arteritis Ask about temporal headache, visual loss or diplopia.

Both may present occasionally with fever, fatigue or weight loss.

Examination

Polymyalgia rheumatica Look for mild tenderness on palpation of the shoulder muscles. Examination of the shoulder joints and neck should be normal.

Giant cell arteritis Look for a tender temporal artery on palpation.

> ⚠ **Giant cell arteritis is an ophthalmological emergency due to the risk of sudden blindness. If the diagnosis is suspected on the grounds of temporal headache and tenderness in patients over the age of 55, the patient should be seen urgently by an ophthalmologist.**

Investigations
- ESR: a result >50 is strongly supportive of the diagnosis of polymyalgia rheumatica. If a borderline raised ESR is obtained, repeat after 48 hours. Do not await the ESR result if there is a strong suspicion of giant cell arteritis.
- Urine: if the ESR is very high, exclude myeloma with urine for Bence–Jones protein.
- TFTs: to exclude hypothyroidism.

Management
- For polymyalgia rheumatica: give prednisolone 10–20 mg daily.
- For giant cell arteritis: urgent referral if suspected, but the starting dose of steroids is 60–80 mg daily.
- For both: stay on the initial dose of prednisolone until the symptoms have come under control, then begin to reduce the daily dose of prednisolone by increments as long as there is no recurrence of symptoms or a significant rise in the ESR.
- Any recurrence of symptoms should prompt an increase in dose for 1 month.
- Most patients are maintained on less than 5 mg daily for the duration of the illness.

> It is not unusual for these patients to require steroids for 2 years or longer, in order to maintain remission of symptoms.

- Beware the risk of osteoporosis in long-term steroid use in the elderly. Use the minimum dose possible. Consider bone densitometry in patients who may be at greatest risk (see osteoporosis, below).

Administration
Give the patient a blue steroid card.

OSTEOPOROSIS

Osteoporosis is most common in postmenopausal women. It is characterised by a decreased bone density due to demineralisation and is responsible for 45 000 hip fractures a year in the UK.

Diagnosis
The condition itself is asymptomatic, but the following put patients at increased risk: • postmenopause • family history of osteoporosis • smoking • lack of exercise • thin build • steroids.

Examination Patients present in the following ways:
- fractured hip or wrist
- back pain which turns out on X-ray to be due to vertebral fracture
- loss of height or dowager's hump, both of which are due to vertebral collapse.

Investigations
- Bone densitometry can detect osteoporosis, but is not yet recommended for screening.
- Blood tests should be normal in osteoporosis.

Management
- Treat the complications of osteoporosis, i.e. fractures.
- The deep bone pain of vertebral collapse usually responds to analgesia and bed rest in 2–4 weeks.
- For the prophylaxis and treatment of osteoporosis, bisphosphonates, e.g. alendronic acid and risedronate, are the drugs of choice. For the prescribing regimen, see the BNF.

Prevention
- Stopping smoking reduces the risk of postmenopausal hip fracture by 25%.
- Regular weight-bearing exercise reduces the risk of postmenopausal hip fracture by up to 50%.
- Five years' use of oestrogen replacement therapy reduces the risk of postmenopausal hip fracture by 50–75% (see hormone replacement therapy, p. 52).
- Reassess the patient's need for steroid therapy.
- Maintain sufficient dietary calcium and vitamin D intake. Supplements (e.g. calcium carbonate up to 40 mmol daily) are only necessary if intake is low.
- Bisphosphonates (see management, above) for treatment of postmenopausal osteoporosis, e.g. alendronic acid 70 mg once weekly, or for prevention of postmenopausal osteoporosis, 5 mg daily.

RHEUMATOID ARTHRITIS

The average GP list of 2000 will have 3–4 rheumatoid arthritis patients. It is three times more common in women. Patients are usually over 40, but may be younger.

Diagnosis
History Ask about:

- Joint pain: symmetrical pain and morning stiffness are very common, especially in the small joints of the hands and feet. The distal interphalangeal joints are usually spared. Swelling of joints often occurs.
- Other symptoms, which include:
  - general malaise
  - weight loss
  - carpal tunnel syndrome
  - tenosynovitis.

Examination Look for:
- Joints which are tender, hot, swollen and painful to move. The proximal interphalangeal, metacarpophalangeal and wrist joints are usually inflamed in the acute phase.
- Carpal tunnel syndrome (see p. 255), which is often associated with rheumatoid arthritis. Tender metatarsophalangeal joints may also be found.

Investigations All suspected cases of rheumatoid arthritis should have ESR or CRP. If these are raised for the patient's age, organise the following:

- FBC.
- Rheumatoid factor: positive in 80% of rheumatoid arthritis patients, but 5% are false-positive results.
- Antinuclear antibody: should be negative to exclude SLE.
- Serum uric acid: should be normal to exclude gout.
- X-ray of the hands and feet: the characteristic appearances of rheumatoid arthritis appear after 6 months of disease.

 It is a mistake not to refer new cases of rheumatoid arthritis at an early stage, since disease-modifying drugs reduce erosive disease and resultant loss of function.

Management

Care of the acute case Refer all patients in whom the diagnosis is suggested or confirmed by the above investigations. Resting acutely inflamed joints reduces pain. Passive movements help prevent deformity.

Drug treatment
- NSAIDs help while awaiting hospital assessment. High-strength NSAIDs at night reduce early morning stiffness and pain, e.g. ibuprofen S/R 800 mg two tablets nocte. Consider a Cox II inhibitor, e.g. rofecoxib 25 mg o.d. for patients at high risk of developing serious gastrointestinal side-effects (see BNF).
- Simple analgesics may be equally effective, e.g. paracetamol.

- If stronger NSAIDs are needed, e.g. indomethacin, H_2 antagonists may be required in addition.
- Acutely inflamed joints can be injected with steroids, e.g. methylprednisolone (see p. 253).

Disease-modifying drugs
- Penicillamine: do an FBC and check urine for protein weekly for 2 months, thereafter monthly.
- Azathioprine: a monthly FBC.
- Sulphasalazine: FBC, C&E and LFT monthly for the first 3 months, thereafter 3-monthly.
- Gold: an FBC and urine for protein and blood before each injection.
- Methotrexate: FBC, C&E and LFT weekly until therapy stabilised, then 3-monthly.

Care of the chronic case The level of help required by the patient depends on the activity of the disease. Not all patients with rheumatoid arthritis have active disease.

- Liaison with the rheumatologist is helpful for prescribing, advice and follow-up.
- Physiotherapy can improve joint mobility and muscle wasting.
- Occupational therapy can address problems with activities of daily living by modification of the home and the provision of walking aids.
- Provide leaflets and support group details.
- Ask the patient to contact Social Services for allowances and benefits, e.g. the orange badge.
- Be aware of potential complications, e.g.:
  – septic arthritis
  – neutropenia
  – drug side-effects
  – atlantoaxial subluxation and quadriplegia in cervical spine involvement
  – dry eyes
  – nodules
  – leg ulcers
  – pulmonary fibrosis
  – peripheral neuropathy.
- Watch for depression and carer stress (see p. 294).
- Consider pain clinic referral.
- Some patients find fish oils and evening primrose oil helpful.
- Advise patients against being overweight.

Try to avoid an unnecessarily gloomy outlook. Many cases follow a mild, remitting course with no long-term disability.

SHOULDER PAIN

Shoulder pain can be a symptom of problems in the neck, such as cervical spondylosis, but is usually caused by either adhesive capsulitis (frozen shoulder) or the rotator cuff syndrome (e.g. supraspinatus tendonitis).

Diagnosis

History Ask about:
- Any history of trauma, such as a fall on the arm.
- Previous episodes of similar problems.
- Neck pain.
- Occupation and handedness: repetitive use of the arm may account for shoulder problems.

Examination Look for:
- Bruising, which may suggest a fractured neck of the humerus, especially in an elderly person following a fall.
- Limitation of movement of the glenohumeral joint, in frozen shoulder.
- The painful arc: pain increases as the shoulder is abducted to about 90°, but reduces again as the arm is raised further above the head. This is a feature of supraspinatus tendonitis.

> **Neck problems often present with shoulder pain.**

Management

- Physiotherapy can be useful for some painful arc syndromes, but is of little value in the treatment of frozen shoulder.
- NSAIDs, if not contraindicated, are useful in reducing pain and inflammation.
- The injection of long-acting corticosteroids into the shoulder joint is useful in the treatment of both supraspinatus tendonitis and frozen shoulder, e.g. methylprednisolone 40 mg with 2% plain lignocaine 2 ml into the glenohumeral joint from either the anterior or the posterior approach (frozen shoulder); or into the subacromial space, using the lateral approach (supraspinatus tendonitis). Warn the patient the pain will get worse over the ensuing 24 hours. If improvement is partial, a second injection is useful.

> ⚠ **Beware the fractured neck of humerus. This is usually more painful initially. Bruising develops over the first 48 hours. Some movement of the glenohumeral joint is often possible.**

TENNIS ELBOW

Tennis elbow is the name usually given to lateral epicondylitis, inflammation of the insertion of the forearm extensor muscles at the elbow.

Diagnosis

History Ask about pain on the outer side of the elbow, especially when gripping. The pain often radiates down the forearm.

Examination Tenderness can be elicited at the point of insertion of the forearm extensor muscles into the lateral epicondyle.

Management
- Tennis elbow can settle spontaneously, but this usually takes several months.
- A short course of NSAIDs can help.
- An injection of e.g. hydrocortisone and local anaesthetic will cure most cases. Using a blue needle inject hydrocortisone 100 mg with 1% lignocaine 1 ml deep into the tender point of the elbow. Warn the patient that the symptoms will worsen over the ensuing 24 hours.
- Ultrasound from the physiotherapist can be an effective alternative.

TENOSYNOVITIS

Tenosynovitis is inflammation of the tendons of the dorsum of the hand or foot. It commonly presents in general practice following repetitive overuse. Occasionally it can occur spontaneously.

Diagnosis

History Ask about pain and tenderness over the tendons, usually of the hand, where they cross the wrist within a synovial sheath. The pain is worsened by movement of the tendon within the sheath.

Examination Look for:
- Swelling. This is a common feature of De Quervain's tenosynovitis (thumb extensors).
- Tenderness and exacerbation of the pain on palpating the affected tendon.

Management
- Rest for 2–3 weeks with immobilisation is often all that is needed. A temporary change of use of the hand may help.
- A short course of NSAIDs can help.

- An injection of hydrocortisone with local anaesthetic may be useful, if the GP is confident in the technique. Refer to a rheumatologist otherwise.
- Referral for surgical decompression is occasionally required, particularly if the above measures are unhelpful and the patient is handicapped by the symptoms.

CARPAL TUNNEL SYNDROME

Carpal tunnel syndrome is the most common cause of paraesthesiae in general practice. The syndrome of pain and tingling in the hand should always raise this possibility.

Diagnosis

History Ask about pain and tingling in the median nerve distribution of the hand. It is usually worse in the mornings and can be relieved temporarily by shaking the hand vigorously.

Examination

> ⚠️ **Wasting of the small muscles of the hand indicates severe nerve compression, and prompt orthopaedic referral for decompression of the carpal tunnel is advised.**

If the symptoms are exacerbated by tapping on the median nerve at the wrist, this is known as a positive Tinnel's sign and is highly suggestive of carpal tunnel syndrome.

Investigations If the diagnosis is in doubt, electromyelographic studies are diagnostic.

Management

- Rest the affected hand. This advice can be supplemented by the provision of a Futura-type wrist splint, or just a plain sling.
- NSAIDs can be useful in mild cases, if not contraindicated.
- Injection of methylprednisolone 40 mg with local anaesthetic under the flexor retinaculum of the wrist, around the median nerve (situated between the radial artery and palmaris longus tendon) can be useful if the GP is confident in this technique. Refer to orthopaedics or rheumatology outpatients otherwise.
- Refer to orthopaedic outpatients for carpal tunnel release if there is no improvement, or if there is wasting of the small muscles of the hand.

GANGLION

A ganglion is a firm, cystic swelling, usually around the dorsum of the wrist or hand. Ganglions can also be found around the ankle. The problem is usually a cosmetic one.

Management
Inform the patient that 50% of all ganglions disappear spontaneously in time. If discomfort or inconvenience is caused by the ganglion it can be treated in a number of ways:

- Aspirate the lump under local anaesthetic using a 21G needle.
- Pierce the ganglion several times with a fine hypodermic needle and press on it gently for several seconds while the contents disperse.

 In both these cases recurrence is possible, so warn the patient of this.

- If the above methods fail, consider referral to orthopaedic outpatients for a formal excision if the patient is troubled by the ganglion.

PARONYCHIA

A paronychia, or whitlow, is a suppurative collection around a fingernail. The pus can easily be seen adjacent to a nail as a white, tense, tender swelling.

Management
- Spray the whitlow with ethyl chloride for 5–10 seconds or until a frost develops.
- Incise through the cuticle into the paronychia using a No. 11 scalpel blade. The pus should be let out and should be seen to drain freely.
- Gently squeeze below the nail bed to 'milk' the pus from the finger. A simple dressing is all that is required.

 If the whitlow has a number of heads it may be herpetic. Acyclovir cream may then be a more appropriate treatment.

- If surrounding cellulitis is a feature, treat with an oral antibiotic, e.g. flucloxacillin.
- If the infection is mild and localised, a topical antibiotic is often sufficient, e.g. fusidic acid.

LOW BACK PAIN

Low back pain is the commonest cause of days lost from work in the UK. Decide first whether the patient is presenting with a new, acute episode of back pain, or a chronic problem.

ACUTE PRESENTATION

The acute onset of lumbar back pain usually follows lifting, and often radiates to the buttock or leg.

Diagnosis

History Ask about: • bladder paralysis symptoms • muscle weakness in the lower limbs • paraesthesiae.

Examination Look for: neurological signs in the lower limbs. Look particularly for weakness of dorsiflection of the ankle and extensor hallucis (L4–L5 prolapse), weakness of the peroneal muscles, toe flexors, calf and tibialis posterior (L5–S1).

Investigations In the elderly with acute back pain, consider ESR and pelvic X-ray (and PSA in men) to exclude malignant disease.

Management

> **Indications for immediate orthopaedic referral are:**
> • **bladder paralysis**
> • **extensive muscle weakness**
> • **objective neurological signs.**

In the absence of neurological signs:

- Advise rest. This may be in bed, but it is not essential to spend 3 days lying on a wooden board. A comfortable position is more important.
- Prescribe analgesics, e.g. co-proxamol 1–2 tablets 6-hourly p.r.n. A laxative helps if opiates are prescribed, e.g. lactulose 10 ml b.d. Diazepam 5 mg t.d.s. is useful, as a muscle relaxant and an anxiolytic, in the short term.
- Follow up if symptoms do not settle in 2–3 days. Repeat the neurological examination.
- For the prevention of further attacks, advise on correct posture, lifting and exercises, and enquire about work-related back strain.

Administration
Sign off work: SC2 for the first week, Med 3 thereafter.

CHRONIC PRESENTATION

 Always think of the possibility of neurological involvement by looking for leg signs and asking about bladder symptoms.

If the acute episode has not settled or repeated acute episodes occur, consider the following: • depression • hidden agenda • carer stress.

Management
- Physical therapy, e.g. physiotherapist, osteopath, chiropractor.
- Orthopaedic referral:
  - MRI scan for prolapsed disc
  - surgery.
- Rheumatology referral: facet joint injection.
- Antidepressants.
- Local back pain sufferers' group.
- Physiotherapist's back school.

KNEE PAIN

After low back pain, knee pain is the second most common orthopaedic problem in general practice.

Diagnosis

History It is useful to divide knee problems into those associated with some trauma to the knee, and those of spontaneous onset.

Without trauma If the pain has been present for some time consider e.g.:
• chondromalacia patellae in the young • osteoarthritis in the elderly.
   If the pain is acute think of: • prepatellar bursitis • septic arthritis • gout.

Prepatellar bursitis can be difficult to distinguish from the rarer septic arthritis. Factors in favour of prepatellar bursitis include:

- an otherwise well patient
- no history of fever
- no limitation of movement of the knee
- the ability to weight-bear.

With trauma If there is no limitation of movement, and the patient can weight-bear, the likely diagnosis is a simple sprain.

Symptoms that suggest damage to the internal structures of the knee include swelling, locking, giving way, inability to weight-bear and an inability to extend the knee fully. Often these symptoms follow a recurring and remitting course.

Examination Watch as the patient undresses and climbs onto the examination couch. This will tell you a lot about the functioning of the knee.

Look for redness, heat and swelling. These suggest the presence of acute inflammation or infection, usually gout, prepatellar bursitis or, occasionally, septic arthritis.

The examination is often normal in chondromalacia patellae, Osgood–Schlatter's disease and minor sprains.

If there is a history of trauma, test the ligaments and cartilages. Holding the lower leg at mid-calf level and with the knee slightly flexed, attempt to bend the knee sideways in each direction in turn. A few degrees of movement is normal, as can be demonstrated on the patient's good knee. Excessive movement suggests a collateral ligament tear. Ask the patient to roll onto his or her front. With the knee flexed to 90°, push down on the foot and rotate the foot in each direction in turn while extending the knee. Acute pain suggests a torn meniscus (McMurray's test).

Management

Chondromalacia patellae
- Conservative management with explanation, analgesics, rest and quadriceps exercises usually suffice.
- Referral for consideration for surgery is rarely needed.

Prepatellar bursitis
- If the inflammation is confined to the patellar area, rest, analgesia and Tubigrip will suffice.
- If there is considerable swelling in front of the knee, aspiration under local anaesthetic will ease the pain by reducing the pressure within the bursa.
- If there is evidence of inflammation extending beyond the area of the patella, antibiotics should be prescribed, e.g. flucloxacillin 250 mg q.d.s.
- If aspiration of the bursa produces pus and there is evidence of cellulitis, consider admitting the patient for surgical drainage and splinting of the knee.

Septic arthritis Admit immediately if this is suspected.

Gout See page 245.

> ⚠️ **Acute knee injuries with swelling require X-rays to exclude a fracture, and aspiration to exclude a haemarthrosis or lipohaemarthrosis. Refer to casualty.**
>
> **In the absence of swelling and if the patient can weight-bear, the acute knee injury can be treated by rest, analgesia, Tubigrip, ice-pack and quadriceps exercises.**

Chronic knee pain
- Chronic traumatic knee pain in a sportsperson can often be helped by a change of footwear.
- Referral to a sports medicine, rheumatology or orthopaedic clinic depends on local specialist interest.
- If the history or examination suggests the presence of either ligament or cartilage damage, consider referral for arthroscopy, especially if quadriceps exercises have not helped.

Osteoarthritis See p. 247.

SPRAINED ANKLE

See management of minor injuries, page 349.

This is a common soft-tissue injury in general practice, usually due to inversion of the ankle, damaging the lateral talofibular ligament. Nearly all soft-tissue sprains settle with rest, followed in severe cases by physiotherapy, but the fractured ankle should be excluded early.

Diagnosis

History Ask about: • falls from a height/down a hole • previous fracture • running/jumping injury • occupation.

Examination Look for:
- tenderness below the lateral malleolus
- tenderness of the fibula above the malleolus (associated with fracture).

> Examine the base of the 5th metatarsal for signs of fracture if the injury is due to a fall, e.g. off the edge of a kerb.

Management
- RICE: **r**est, **i**ce, **c**ompression (Tubigrip), **e**levation.
- Mobilise gently after 24 hours.
- Refer more severe sprains, e.g. sports injuries, for physiotherapy early.

> Pain, swelling and bruising get worse over the first 24 hours in the
> sprained ankle. Use ice for 10–15 minutes at a time.

Referral Referral for an orthopaedic opinion is appropriate if the patient does
not improve to the point of returning to work after physiotherapy.

Administration
Self-certificate SC2 (up to 7 days).

PAINFUL HEEL (PLANTAR FASCIITIS)

Plantar fasciitis causes chronic pain under the heel with no history of trauma.
There is usually a tender spot just in front of the bony part of the heel. The
condition is self-limiting and usually resolves spontaneously after several months.

Diagnosis

Differential diagnosis
- Plantar wart: can usually be seen.
- Fracture calcaneum: follows quite severe trauma.
- Sever's disease (osteochondritis of the calcaneum): tender at the tendo-
  Achilles insertion.

Management
- Plantar fasciitis may respond to a short course of NSAIDs with rest.
- An injection of hydrocortisone with local anaesthetic can be performed.
  Warn the patient that the symptoms will get temporarily worse over the
  ensuing 24 hours. Using an orange needle on a 5-ml syringe inject 1% plain
  lignocaine 2 ml with hydrocortisone 100 mg or methylprednisolone 40 mg
  deep into the tender spot. This can be repeated two or three times at
  intervals of 3 weeks.

Administration
As for shoulder injection (see p. 253).

INGROWING TOENAIL

An ingrowing toenail is a spike of toenail growing into the nail-fold, causing
pain and infection.

Management

Conservative management Show the patient how to elevate the nail edge. Recommend that this is done after a long soak in a warm bath. A nail file or other blunt instrument can be used. A pledget of cotton wool can be pushed under the elevated nail. This should be done daily for a week or so.

If the nail edge looks infected, prescribe an antibiotic, e.g. oral flucloxacillin, for 5 days.

Surgical management
- Nail edge excision can be performed in general practice if the GP is confident in the technique. Otherwise, refer to a surgical podiatrist or orthopaedic outpatients.
- Consider Zadik's procedure (bilateral wedge excision) for recurrent cases.

Prevention

Encourage square nail-cutting, i.e. advise the patient to avoid trying to cut the nail with a curve at the edges. This allows the edges to grow free of the end of the toe without digging in.

SURGERY

PAEDIATRIC PROBLEMS

HERNIA AND HYDROCELE

These usually present in the first year of life as a swelling in the groin. They may present after an episode of crying or coughing.

> ⚠️ **An obstructed hernia is tender and it is impossible to palpate above it, unlike other causes of a groin swelling:**
> • hydrocele • incompletely descended testicle • inguinal lymphadenopathy • groin abscess.

Referral to a paediatric surgeon is indicated. Admit to hospital any patient with a suspected obstructed hernia.

UNDESCENDED TESTES

Incompletely descended testes are seen in 0.5–0.7% of boys at 1 year of age.
Referral to a paediatric surgeon is indicated at the first presentation, regardless of age or degree of maldescent.

PHIMOSIS

The foreskin is usually non-retractile until the age of 5 years. A tight meatus and spraying urinary stream may suggest the need for circumcision.
Recurrent balanitis is best treated with improved hygiene and intermittent oral antibiotics. Circumcision is indicated for persistent cases.

UMBILICAL GRANULOMA

Pyogenic granuloma of the umbilical remnant is a common problem at the 6–8-week check.
The application of silver nitrate, or alternatively ligation, are effective, simple measures.

UMBILICAL HERNIAE

The true umbilical hernia, or protruding umbilicus, should not be referred as surgery is not usually required. Strangulation is very rare in these cases.
Supra-umbilical and epigastric herniae should be referred, as trapping of bowel or omentum is more common.

INTUSSUSCEPTION

Intussusception is most common under the age of 2 years and presents as severe colic, vomiting and pallor, often with blood in the stool.

Admission to hospital is clearly indicated.

LEG PROBLEMS

Some normal conditions cause parental anxiety. These include: bow legs, flat feet, knock knees, in- and out-toeing and walking on tiptoes. As long as there is no pain or limp, and the examination reveals a full range of pain-free movement, the parents should be reassured that all is well.

LIMP

A persistent limp is usually pathological and referral to an orthopaedic surgeon is indicated. The acute onset of a limp with pain in the hip requires an urgent orthopaedic opinion, to exclude septic arthritis and slipped femoral epiphysis.

BREAST LUMPS

All breast lumps cause anxiety in the patient until a firm diagnosis is made.

Management

Refer patients with breast lumps to a surgeon with an interest in treating breast cancer.

Examination of the patient may reveal a softish lump that is neither fixed nor tethered to muscle or skin. The patient can then be reassured that there are no obvious features to suggest malignancy, prior to referral.

Aspiration If the lump feels soft or cystic it is worth attempting to aspirate it. This is easy.

- Fix the lump between finger and thumb of the left hand, having cleaned the skin with an alcohol wipe.
- Pierce the lump with a green needle on a 10-ml syringe and withdraw the plunger.
- If the breast lump contains fluid, the syringe will start to fill. When no more fluid can be aspirated, remove the needle.

- If the lump has disappeared to palpation it was a benign cyst and the patient need not be referred. However, always send the fluid for cytology to double-check.

LUMPY BREASTS

Anxiety about cancer in a woman with lumpy or large breasts poses a difficult problem. If normal on clinical examination, mammography may be useful.

PAINFUL BREASTS

Cyclical mastalgia in the absence of lumps can be treated by:

- reassurance that there are no lumps
- evening primrose oil, 2–3 capsules t.d.s. (only available OTC)
- frusemide 40 mg daily for premenstrual fluid retention.

GALLSTONES

The symptoms of gallstones are often confused with gastric problems. Most gallstones are asymptomatic.

Diagnosis

History Ask about: • right hypochondrial pain • anorexia • nausea • jaundice • pale stools and dark urine.

Examination Look for: • tenderness in the right hypochondrium, which is worse on deep inspiration • jaundice.

Investigations
- Upper abdominal ultrasound usually shows gallstones if present.
- Request LFTs if the patient is jaundiced, to determine whether obstruction of the common bile duct has occurred.

Differential diagnosis
- Upper abdominal pain: gastric causes, e.g. gastritis, duodenal ulcer, reflux.
- Severe pain with constitutional upset: e.g. acute pancreatitis, perforation.
- Obstructive jaundice: e.g. tumour.

Management

Acute
- Pain relief, e.g. diclofenac 75 mg i.m., followed by e.g. co-proxamol, 2 tablets, 4–6-hourly.

- Advise a low-fat diet.
- Arrange an ultrasound routinely.

 In the severe attack with constitutional upset (vomiting, pyrexia, tachycardia), acute admission to hospital is necessary.

- If jaundice is present, with obstructive LFT changes, discuss with the on-call surgeon regarding admission for urgent ERCP.

Chronic
- In patients with recurrent attacks of acute pain and with ultrasound evidence of stones, referral for surgery is indicated.
- Occasionally the specialist may advise medical treatment, e.g. deoxycholic acid.

HERNIAE IN THE GROIN

Inguinal herniae are usually found by the patient as a painless swelling in the groin. Occasionally they present in the early stages as groin pain. Femoral herniae tend to be more painful.

Diagnosis
Examination
- Examine the patient standing up.
- Look for a swelling with a cough impulse.
- Is the swelling reducible?
- Can it be controlled by pressure on the internal inguinal ring (above and lateral to the pubic tubercle)? If so, it is an indirect inguinal hernia.
- A femoral hernia is above and medial to the pubic tubercle. In practice this makes it feel as though it is sitting on the pubic bone.
- If a swelling in the groin is due to a hydrocele, it is usually possible to palpate above the swelling.

Management

 Femoral and indirect inguinal herniae can strangulate, causing abdominal pain, abdominal swelling, vomiting and absolute constipation (obstruction). Give i.v. pain relief and admit the patient directly to hospital.

Referral Femoral and indirect inguinal herniae need referring for elective surgery.

Conservative management Where the patient is unsuitable for surgery, or the hernia is an easily reducible inguinal hernia, some relief can be provided by the provision of a truss. This is prescribable on the NHS.

SCROTAL SWELLINGS

The most common causes of a swelling in the scrotum are an inguinoscrotal hernia or hydrocele, followed by an epididymal cyst.

A sebaceous cyst of the scrotal skin may be described as a scrotal swelling. Testicular tumours are rare.

Diagnosis

History Ask about pain in the scrotum. The following are painless:
• inguinoscrotal hernia • hydrocele • epididymal cyst. Otherwise, see testicular pain, page 269.

A history of trauma suggests either a secondary hydrocele or haematocele.

Examination
• Examine the patient standing.
• If you cannot palpate above the swelling, it is an inguinoscrotal hernia.
• If you can palpate above the swelling and it is above the testicle, it is either an epididymal cyst or a varicocele. An epididymal cyst will transilluminate. A varicocele feels like a bag of worms.
• A hydrocele is usually large and tense and transilluminates easily. The testicle cannot be palpated as it is within the hydrocele.
• A sebaceous cyst is superficial and confined to the scrotal skin.
• Testicular tumours cause enlargement of a testicle.

Investigations If you are in any doubt about the diagnosis, particularly with regard to excluding a possible tumour of the testis, request a scrotal ultrasound scan.

Management
• Sebaceous cyst: reassure.
• Hydrocele: aspirate (see below).
• All others: refer.

Aspiration of a hydrocele
Only if the GP has the confidence to perform the procedure correctly. Otherwise, refer.

- Avoid the testicle by locating it with transillumination.
- Clean the skin with an alcohol wipe.
- Insert a green needle on a 20-ml syringe and draw off as much fluid as possible.
- Always palpate the testicle afterwards to exclude a tumour of the testis as a cause of the hydrocele.
- Repeat the procedure as necessary. Frequent recurrences need surgical treatment.

TESTICULAR PAIN

The most common presentation of testicular pain in general practice is mild and transient, and a cause is often not found.

Diagnosis
History

> ⚠ **Severe pain in the testicle suggests torsion or acute epididymo-orchitis. Nausea and vomiting often occur in torsion. Torsion is extremely rare over the age of 25.**

- A recent history of cystitis, prostatitis or prostatectomy suggests epididymo-orchitis, as does a history of STI or urethral discharge.
- Mumps may be complicated by orchitis.

Examination
- In torsion the genitalia are often too tender to examine.
- In epididymo-orchitis there may be red skin over the infection, and the most tender part is often felt to be above the testicle.
- In both torsion and epididymo-orchitis there may be a scrotal swelling due to oedema or inflammation.
- Examination of the painful testicle is often normal, in which case mild epididymitis is probably the cause.
- Other possible causes of pain in the testicle include:
  - ureteric calculi
  - inguinoscrotal hernia
  - groin strain
  - malignancy.

Management

Admit all cases of severe pain as possible torsion.

In less severe cases, where the examination is normal, it is wise to wait and see what happens with time. Most cases resolve spontaneously without any treatment. Those that do not settle may be helped by prescribing an anti-inflammatory, such as ibuprofen 400 mg t.d.s.

If there are signs suggesting epididymo-orchitis, such as erythema and fever, take an MSU (and urethral swab for gonococcus, if appropriate) and treat with a broad-spectrum antibiotic such as ciprofloxacin 500 mg b.d. for 5 days. Consider referral to the genitourinary medicine clinic.

ANAL FISSURE

Diagnosis

History and examination The patient experiences sharp anal pain on defaecation. An anal fissure can mimic some of the symptoms of piles, but appears as a sore-looking crack in the skin at the anal margin. If present, an anal fissure often makes digital rectal examination extremely painful.

Management
- The patient should avoid constipation, with a high-fibre diet ± a bulking laxative.
- Stool-softeners often allow the fissure to heal.
- Xyloproct or Proctosedyl suppositories, inserted before passing a stool, will allow the bowels to be opened less painfully.
- Glyceryl trinitrate cream applied to the anal margins helps relieve sphincter muscle spasm pain.
- The anal fissure that is severe, or will not heal with suppositories and laxatives, may require surgical referral for an anal stretch or partial internal sphincterotomy.

HAEMORRHOIDS

Piles, or haemorrhoids, are one of the commonest causes of rectal bleeding.

Diagnosis

History Ask about:

- The nature of the rectal bleeding. With haemorrhoids this is usually bright red, painless and often drips into the toilet pan or is seen on the toilet paper. It is not mixed with the stool, but more often streaked on the surface of the stool.
- Anal irritation.
- Prolapsed or external piles, which can be felt by the patient as lumps outside the anus. These may be confused with anal skin tags.

Examination Look for:

- External piles and skin tags, which are obvious on inspection of the anal margin. Thrombosed piles are acutely tender, hard, purple lumps.
- Internal piles, which can be seen on passing a proctoscope and look like small purple bulges about 4 cm (1½ in.) inside the anal margin.
- A mass higher up in the rectum, by performing a digital rectal examination.
- An abdominal mass, by palpating the abdomen.

Investigations Investigations are unnecessary for piles.

> ⚠ **Caution is needed in attributing new rectal bleeding to piles in patients aged over 40. Consider referral for colonoscopy in all cases, as large bowel cancer and piles are both common and can coexist.**

Management

- Advise the patient to avoid constipation, straining at stool and sitting for too long.
- A laxative and/or a bulking agent, e.g. ispaghula husk granules, often help to prevent the piles worsening.
- Proctosedyl or Xyloproct ointment or suppositories are useful for anal irritation or soreness, and also for healing an anal fissure.
- Injection of piles is easy and will symptomatically cure about 50% of cases. This can be done in general practice or by referral to surgical outpatients.
- Consider referral for haemorrhoidectomy for third-degree piles, painful piles, heavy bleeding or failure of phenol injection.

PROSTATISM

See page 70.

VARICOSE VEINS AND ULCERATION

Varicose veins and ulcers are ubiquitous problems in general practice.

VARICOSE VEINS

Diagnosis

History Ask about: ● pain and aching ● appearance ● phlebitis ● ulceration.

Examination Look for signs of ulceration, varicose eczema, bleeding and thrombophlebitis.

Management
- Advise elevation of the legs, when possible.
- Advise weight loss if appropriate.
- Advise support stockings, e.g. class one or two thigh-length graduated stockings (available on prescription).
- Referral for ligation and multiple avulsion should be considered if the patient is considerably troubled or handicapped by the complications of varicose veins. Patients requesting 'cosmetic' varicose vein surgery should be referred privately.

VARICOSE ULCERATION
See page 358.

APPENDICITIS

Appendicitis presents about two or three times a year to the GP with the average list of 2000 patients. Pain in the right iliac fossa due to other causes is far more frequent.

Diagnosis

History Pain in the abdomen is often the first symptom to be noticed in appendicitis. It is usually in the right iliac fossa, having moved there from the centre of the abdomen over the preceding 24 hours. In the early stages this is often the only symptom and can be quite severe before the other symptoms (e.g. vomiting, constipation) arise.

A concomitant URTI with abdominal pain suggests mesenteric adenitis in a child.

Diarrhoea is unusual in appendicitis, and suggests gastroenteritis.

Examination Patients with appendicitis requiring hospital treatment will be mildly pyrexial, and tender in the right iliac fossa, with guarding and rebound tenderness and quiet bowel sounds. They will also usually have a tachycardia, halitosis and dry lips.

The milder case may only have slight tenderness in the abdomen and no other symptoms.

Investigations An FBC will show a raised neutrophil count in appendicitis. In cases requiring hospital admission on clinical grounds there is no indication for the GP to do a blood test first.

Management

The management of severe acute appendicitis is hospital admission and appendicectomy. If there is doubt in the GP's mind as to the severity of the case, it should be discussed with the surgical registrar.

In mild cases it is acceptable to treat in general practice. If appendicitis is suspected but the patient is not unwell, it is reasonable to treat with metronidazole and a cephalosporin in conjunction with some mild analgesia. It is important to review the patient for signs of worsening over 24–48 hours.

Grumbling appendix Repeated attacks of appendicitis that settle down with conservative measures are due to a 'grumbling appendix'. Referral to surgical outpatients is advised for consideration for an interval appendicectomy, i.e. between the attacks.

PERIODS OF INCAPACITY AFTER SURGERY

Times off work following surgery vary depending on surgical complications, patient health and fitness and occupation, but as a rule of thumb the following advice can be given to patients:

- Vasectomy: 2 days.
- Cholecystectomy: 2 weeks.
- Hernia repair: 2 weeks.
- Hysterectomy: 6 weeks.
- Caesarian section: 6 weeks.
- Coronary bypass: 2 months.
- Hip replacement: 2 months.

NEUROLOGY

DIZZINESS

Many different sensations are described as dizziness. These include light-headedness, muzziness and faintness. First decide whether the patient is experiencing true vertigo, which is a subjective sensation of rotation, either of the patient or the surroundings. It is often accompanied by nausea, and nystagmus is a common finding.

Causes of true vertigo
- Common: labyrinthitis, benign positional vertigo.
- Rare:
  - brainstem stroke/TIA
  - vertebrobasilar insufficiency
  - Ménière's disease
  - acoustic neuroma
  - multiple sclerosis.

Causes of other types of dizziness • Infections, e.g. flu-like illnesses and URTIs • anxiety and depression (see pp. 294 and 296) • syncope (see funny turns, p. 157).

LABYRINTHITIS

Diagnosis
Labyrinthitis is the commonest cause of true vertigo in general practice. Apart from nausea and vomiting and possible nystagmus, there are no other symptoms or signs. Features such as hearing loss or tinnitus suggest Ménière's disease or acoustic neuroma. Focal neurological signs suggest an intracerebral pathology.

Management
- Reassure the patient that the condition is not due to a tumour, is common and that it completely resolves.
- Explain that the symptoms will be severe for 2–3 days and that total recovery is usually within 6 weeks. Labyrinthitis is probably due to inflammation of the inner ear and it is often recurrent.
- If symptomatic treatment is required, prescribe prochlorperazine 5 mg p.o. t.d.s. or give 12.5 mg i.m. if the patient is vomiting.
- Advise patients not to drive until symptoms are adequately controlled. Group 2 license holders are banned from driving for at least a year after symptoms have been controlled if they have suffered uncontrolled, disabling giddiness.

> Referral to a neurologist or ENT consultant is indicated if the diagnosis is in doubt, or if other features suggest an alternative diagnosis. Failure to make a full recovery in the expected time scale should also suggest the need for specialist investigation.

HEADACHE

Ninety per cent of headaches are tension headaches; 8–12% of the population have migraines. It is estimated that 0.004% of headaches are due to serious pathology.

Diagnosis

Causes of headache

- Common:
  - tension headache
  - associated with URTI
  - migraine
  - depression.
- Rare:
  - tumour
  - subarachnoid haemorrhage
  - subdural haemorrhage
  - meningitis
  - giant cell arteritis.

> Often the cause of a headache cannot be neatly classified. As long as there are no features of serious disease (see below), reassurance and a 'wait and see' approach are reasonable.

Examination • BP • fundi • neck muscles • cervical spine movements • temporal arteries.

Indicators of more serious disease in headache
- Sudden onset.
- New, severe headache.
- Progressively worsening headache.
- Onset of headaches after the age of 50.
- Altered level of consciousness.
- Recent head injury.
- Abnormal physical findings, especially focal neurology.
- Meningism.
- Tender temporal arteries.

Management

Referral Indications for referral are:
- any of the above serious features
- failure to improve with adequate treatment
- uncertain diagnosis if the headaches are disabling
- patient's insistence.

TENSION HEADACHE

The features of tension headaches are: • chronic, frequent and recurrent
• moderately severe • generalised • described as a tight band of pressure
• absence of nausea generally • scalp tenderness in places.
Examination is otherwise normal.

Management

Reassurance, relaxation and analgesics are often all that are necessary (see anxiety, p. 296).

MIGRAINE

The features of migraines are:
- They are usually unilateral, severe, aching, pulsating and worse on activity.
- Nausea, vomiting, photophobia and phonophobia can occur.
- They last from 4 to 72 hours and are recurrent.
- Visual disturbance occurs in 20%.

Examination should be normal.

Management

- Advise the patient to avoid precipitants, e.g. caffeine, alcohol, tiredness, stress, dehydration, missed meals, combined oral contraceptive (see p. 3).
- Analgesics are the first line of treatment, e.g. paracetamol, codeine, dihydrocodeine and NSAIDs.
- The NSAID folfenamic acid is licensed specifically for migraine.
- Anti-emetics are also often required, e.g. metoclopramide.
- Combinations of analgesics and anti-emetics are available e.g. Migraleve.
- A 5-HT agonist, such as sumatriptan 50–100 mg p.o. or 6 mg by autoinjector or 20 mg (one spray) intranasally, is an effective alternative, but is expensive.

Prophylaxis
For the patient experiencing frequent repeat attacks, say ≥ 2 attacks per month, consider the need for prophylaxis, e.g. propranolol 40 mg b.d. or t.d.s. or pizotifen 1.5–3 mg nocte or a tricyclic antidepressant (even when the patient is not obviously depressed).

FACIAL PAIN

The common causes of facial pain in general practice are: • trigeminal neuralgia • sinusitis • dental infection or impaction • temporomandibular joint dysfunction • ear infections • mumps • submandibular lymphadenopathy • migraine.

A rare, but important, cause of facial pain is temporal arteritis.

> Often the cause of a patient's facial pain cannot be neatly categorised. Patients with depression can present with a facial pain that is probably psychosomatic (see p. 299).

TRIGEMINAL NEURALGIA

Diagnosis
The patient complains of severe, stabbing or burning pain in the distribution of one or more branches of the fifth cranial nerve. It is unilateral and made worse on lightly touching the skin or on exposure to cold wind.

Management
- Simple analgesics are often all that is required, as most cases get better within a few weeks.
- Carbamazepine 100 mg t.d.s., increased to 200 mg t.d.s. according to response, is useful in more severe pain.
- Treatment of depression, if present, may be indicated (see p. 294).
- Referral to a neurologist may be indicated if the above measures fail. Some patients benefit from injection or surgical resection of the affected trigeminal nerve branch.

TEMPOROMANDIBULAR JOINT DYSFUNCTION

Diagnosis
The patient complains of pain in front of the ear, exacerbated by eating and often accompanied by clicking.

Management
- Reassurance that the condition is benign and temporary is often all that is required.
- Advising patients to alter their bite by chewing on the other side of the mouth is useful.

- Advise patients to avoid very chewy food, e.g. hard crusts.
- NSAIDs are sometimes required for more painful episodes.
- Severe cases, involving locking of the jaw, may need referral to a faciomaxillary surgeon.

OTHER CAUSES

Sinusitis
See page 222.

Dental infection or impaction
Refer the patient to his or her dentist.

Ear pain
See page 218.

Mumps
See page 209.

Submandibular lymphadenopathy
See page 224.

Migraine
See page 278.

Temporal arteritis
See page 248.

BELL'S PALSY

Bell's palsy is the idiopathic palsy of the facial nerve (VII) resulting in a unilateral facial weakness or paralysis. It may be preceded by pain behind the ear, but usually presents as a painless facial paralysis.

Diagnosis

Examination
- Exclude geniculate herpes by looking for vesicles in the ear and mouth.
- Make sure that the patient can close the eye on the affected side, to avoid corneal abrasion (see below).
- Examination of the other cranial nerves should be normal.

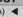

> ⚠️ **A CVA** involving the upper motor neurone of the seventh cranial nerve can give a similar facial weakness. In this case, however, the patient should still be able to raise the eyebrow on the affected side. This is not possible in Bell's palsy.

Management

- 65% of cases recover completely within a few weeks, with or without treatment. Others take longer.
- Prednisolone 40 mg daily for 1 week, reducing to zero over a further 3 weeks, may speed the recovery.
- For patients unable to close the affected eye, prescribe an artificial tear solution, such as hypromellose eyedrops, and advise that they tape the eyelid down at night. This helps to prevent corneal scarring.

> Partial improvement by day 10 and a young age at onset are good prognostic indicators.

- Consider referral to a neurologist if the diagnosis is in doubt.
- For patients with residual paresis, contractures or facial asymmetry, the opinion of a plastic surgeon should be sought.

CEREBROVASCULAR ACCIDENT (CVA)

The GP with the average list of 2000 patients will see 3–4 strokes per year and about one transient ischaemic attack (TIA).

> An acute stroke is defined as a rapid onset of clinically evident focal cerebral deficit lasting more than 24 hours, with no obvious cause.

Diagnosis

Examination

- Neurological examination, as appropriate.
- Check for cardiac arrhythmias (e.g. atrial fibrillation) and carotid bruits.
- Blood pressure.

Investigations
- Bloods for FBC, ESR, U&E, glucose and cholesterol/lipids.
- CXR.
- ECG.

Management

Referral In general all patients with acute strokes should be considered for admission to hospital. Early CT scanning, thrombolysis or anticoagulation and antiplatelet therapy can all help prevent further attacks. One can wait 24 hours before deciding on admission, since improvement may be rapid (see TIAs, p. 283).

However, patients whose quality of life is poor, such as some severely disabled nursing-home residents, should not be admitted as they stand to gain little or nothing from this action.

Prescribing Start the patient on aspirin 150 mg o.d. and a statin (see p. 145).

Management of the patient with disability
- Check that Social Services support is adequate.
- Be alert for signs of depression (see p. 294) and carer stress.
- Check that Attendance Allowance is being claimed, that the Driver and Vehicle Licensing Agency has been informed, and that a disabled parking permit has been applied for, if appropriate.
- Refer the patient for speech therapy, if needed.
- Rehabilitation may also be necessary, e.g. physiotherapy and occupational therapy. Consider domiciliary services.

Secondary prevention of stroke
Check:

- life-style factors (see p. 138)
- BP (see p. 138)
- Smoking status (see p. 138)
- cholesterol (see p. 145)
- blood glucose (see p. 98).

Prognosis There is a 10% annual risk of a serious vascular event after a stroke, e.g. a further stroke, MI or death. This risk is reduced by 25% with the use of aspirin.

Be encouraging and optimistic with stroke patients about their functional recovery, which can be slow. Little improvement at 6 weeks, however, carries a poor prognosis, with permanent disability likely.

Patients can resume driving after at least 1 month following a stroke if recovery is satisfactory. Patients should inform the Driver and Vehicle Licensing Agency after this time if there is anything more than minor limb dysfunction.

TRANSIENT ISCHAEMIC ATTACK (TIA)

- Full recovery of all the neurological signs should occur within 24 hours.
- Examine the patient for signs of cardiac arrhythmias (see p. 158) and carotid bruits.
- Check bloods for FBC, ESR, U&E, glucose and cholesterol.
- Request a CXR and ECG.
- Start the patient on aspirin 150 mg daily and a statin (see p. 145).

> Serious consideration should be given to the referral of the patient to a vascular surgeon for carotid Doppler studies. A significant number of patients with a TIA have carotid stenosis, which is treatable by carotid endarterectomy. Not all patients in this group have a carotid bruit on examination.

TREMOR

Benign essential tremor is very common in general practice. Other common causes of tremor in general practice are Parkinson's syndrome, anxiety and thyrotoxicosis. Rare causes include the cerebellar disorders.

Diagnosis

Categories of tremor
There are essentially three:

- positional tremors, e.g. essential, anxiety and thyrotoxicosis tremors
- the resting tremor of Parkinson's syndrome
- the intention tremor of cerebellar disorders.

POSITIONAL TREMOR

An essential tremor is a fine, rapid tremor, especially of the hands, exacerbated by holding the arms outstretched. No other features of Parkinson's syndrome should be present (see p. 284).

Pathological causes of this type of tremor are extremely rare but can be excluded by taking a history and checking blood tests for: • alcohol excess • thyrotoxicosis • drugs (e.g. salbutamol) • carbon monoxide poisoning.

Management

The main drug used in the treatment of benign essential tremor is propranolol 40 mg b.d., increasing at weekly intervals, according to the response, up to 80–160 mg daily.

Referral to a neurologist is unlikely to be necessary, but should be considered if the symptoms are worsening despite adequate doses of a beta blocker.

RESTING TREMOR

See Parkinson's syndrome, below.

INTENTION TREMOR

Refer all cases of intention tremor, as a cerebellar tumour is a possible cause. Other features may include: • nystagmus • ataxia • past-pointing • falls.

PARKINSON'S SYNDROME

One per cent of people over 60 years of age have Parkinson's syndrome.

Diagnosis

History Ask about: • shaking • falls • stiffness • slowness • decreased handwriting size.

Examination Look for the triad of: • tremor • rigidity • bradykinesia.
Common features are: • a resting, pill-rolling tremor • reduced arm swinging when walking, with festinant (hesitating) gait • decreased facial expression • cog-wheel rigidity • small handwriting.

In the early stages of Parkinson's syndrome the diagnosis can be difficult to make. It is perfectly acceptable to wait and see if symptoms worsen, as the diagnosis will become obvious with time.

Management

- Stop, if possible, any drugs which may be causing Parkinsonism, e.g. phenothiazines and butyrophenones.
- L-Dopa with a dopa decarboxylase inhibitor (Sinemet or Madopar) is the main drug in the treatment of Parkinson's syndrome. It is best in patients with marked bradykinesia. Start with the lowest dose, i.e. 100 mg o.d. of L-dopa equivalent. Increase the dose over several weeks to 400–800 mg daily in divided doses, until a good therapeutic effect is achieved.
  - Side-effects include nausea, vomiting, anorexia, postural hypotension and agitation.
- Anticholinergics, e.g. benzhexol, can be added if necessary. They are best in patients with rigidity and tremor. Start with 2 mg b.d., increasing to 5 mg b.d.
  - Side-effects include blurred vision, dry mouth, constipation, palpitations, urinary retention and glaucoma.
- Referral to a neurologist should be considered if the patient is young, if the diagnosis is uncertain, for failure of the above therapy and problematical side-effects, and for a decreasing effect of therapy after initial success.
- General support can be usefully provided in general practice. Consider physiotherapy and occupational therapy, Social Services, Attendance Allowance and day hospital. Emotional support and carer support are also important.
- Look out for depression (see p. 294) and dementia (see p. 304).

FALLS

Falls are common in the elderly and have a multitude of possible causes:

- Visual: cataract, macular degeneration, refractive error.
- Environmental: loose carpet, steps.
- Musculoskeletal: Parkinson's syndrome, arthritis.
- Drugs: postural hypotension.
- Cardiac: arrhythmia, heart block.
- Neurological: TIA, epilepsy.
- Circulatory: vertebrobasilar insufficiency.

Diagnosis

History Ask patients to describe what happens during a fall:

- Do they remember falling?
- Do they get any warning that they are going to fall?
- Are there any associated symptoms, e.g. palpitations?
- Take a drug history.

Examination
- Examine BP sitting and standing, to look for a postural drop.
- Observe the gait.
- Auscultate the heart.
- Look for any gross neurological signs.

Investigations ECG, if heart block or other cardiac causes are suspected.

Management
If the cause can be categorised, refer to the specific page, as necessary, for:
• decreased vision (p. 239) • osteoarthritis (p. 247) • Parkinson's syndrome
(p. 284) • loss of consciousness (p. 157) • dizziness (p. 276) • epilepsy (see below).

Often the cause cannot immediately be found. Advise the patient to use a stick or frame if appropriate. Physiotherapy or day hospital referral may be helpful. Referral to a physician with an interest in the elderly may be indicated in frequent, undiagnosed falls.

EPILEPSY

The GP with the average list of 2000 patients might expect to have about eight patients with epilepsy.

Diagnosis
History
- Suspect epilepsy after a seizure, i.e. uncontrolled nervous activity, with or without a convulsion or loss of consciousness.
- Take a careful history, from witnesses if possible. Particular reference should be made to rigidity, shaking, loss of consciousness, incontinence, tongue-biting and post-ictal drowsiness.
- Focal seizures and absence attacks are also included in the diagnosis.

Differential diagnosis
- Syncope: preceding faintness, pallor, sweating, rapid and full recovery (see p. 157).
- TIA: dysphasia, paresis or other temporary loss of function (see p. 283).

Management
Initial management

All patients suspected of having epilepsy should be referred after a single seizure.

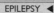

Refer to a neurologist with an interest in epilepsy, if possible, and suggest that the patient is accompanied by a witness to the attacks.

Management during a fit
- Ensure the airway is clear and that the patient is breathing.
- Check the pulse at the carotid.
- Put the patient in the left lateral position.
- Administer rectal diazepam, 10 mg (5 mg in children).

Admit the patient to hospital if:

- **this is the first fit**
- **the cause is not yet known**
- **it is a prolonged fit**
- **there are poor social circumstances**
- **the patient has a head injury**
- **there are any residual problems, e.g. paresis.**

Counselling after a diagnosis of epilepsy has been made

Safety Advise the patient to avoid heights, e.g. ladders, and to swim only under supervision in shallow water.

Driving Epileptics are banned from driving on an ordinary licence for 1 year after their last fit. A licence is granted if the convulsions have been solely nocturnal for at least 3 years. There is a total ban on vocational licences. After the first suspected fit, advise the patient not to drive until he or she has seen the neurologist.

First aid and seizure control Give advice to relatives about first aid during a seizure and prescribe rectal diazepam 10 mg to be used in the event of further fits.

Medic Alert bracelet This is advisable for all epileptics.

Anticonvulsant drug interactions Check whether the patient is taking any drugs that may interfere with anticonvulsants, especially the contraceptive pill. The effectiveness of both combined oral contraceptives and progestogen-only pills is reduced by carbamazepine, phenytoin, phenobarbitone and primidone. Use 50 μg oestrogen pills or an alternative method (see p. 6).

Drug side-effects
- Carbamazepine: drowsiness, dizziness, headache, gastrointestinal upset.

- Phenytoin: acne, hirsutism, gum hyperplasia.
- Sodium valproate: weight gain, hair loss, nausea, ataxia, tremor.

Preconception counselling Advise female patients that they will need to be referred to their neurologist if they are contemplating getting pregnant.

Breast-feeding All anticonvulsants, except barbiturates, can be prescribed to breast-feeding mothers.

Prescription charge exemption Patients with epilepsy are exempt from prescription charges.

Avoidance of triggers Alcohol, tiredness and flashing lights are the common triggers for seizures in susceptible patients.

Disease monitoring
- If fits are still occurring, increase the dose of the first-line anticonvulsant until the fits are controlled without unwanted side-effects.
- Aim for therapeutic drug levels with:
  - carbamazepine 20–50 µmol/l
  - phenytoin 40–80 µmol/l.
- If the fits are not controlled with the maximum dose of the first-line drug, refer patients back to their consultant.
- If the fits are controlled, see the patient 6–12-monthly. Consider:
  - side-effects
  - drug levels, if appropriate (fits, side-effects, change of dose or starting a drug which interacts)
  - counselling, as above.

MULTIPLE SCLEROSIS

The average GP's list of 2000 patients will contain one or two patients with multiple sclerosis.

The mean age of onset is 35 years, with a range, commonly, of between 20 and 40 years of age.

Diagnosis

History There is a wide variety of presenting symptoms in multiple sclerosis. These are due to acute episodes of demyelination, and common examples are:

- optic neuritis: partial or complete loss of vision, with or without pain
- diplopia
- nystagmus
- vertigo
- weakness or paraesthesia in a limb (see dermatomes, p. 380)

- ataxia
- an extensor plantar reflex
- diminished vibration sense
- loss of abdominal reflexes.

The symptoms commonly develop in a matter of hours or days and disappear over weeks.

 A careful history of past symptoms may reveal a previous episode of possible demyelination, making the diagnosis more likely.

Examination Examination of the relevant part of the nervous system may reveal objective signs. A full neurological examination would be very time-consuming for a GP, but may demonstrate further signs of demyelination.

Physical examination is often normal in the initial stages of multiple sclerosis. It is a sad but well-recognised phenomenon that patients with their first episode of demyelination are often labelled as hysterical.

Management
All suspected cases should be referred for a neurological opinion.

Prognosis Fifteen years from presentation, approximately one-third of patients with multiple sclerosis will be severely disabled, but another third will be unrestricted by disability.

The average life expectancy is 25 years from presentation.

Long-term care
- Close communication with the patient's neurologist is important, especially if the patient relapses or deteriorates.
- Physiotherapy is useful for contractures, immobility and poor posture.
- Occupational therapy helps with the activities of daily living.
- A social worker can help with employment matters, allowances and re-housing.
- For the treatment of spasticity, consider physiotherapy. Treatment with baclofen or dantrolene may be useful.
- Flexion deformities also may be helped by physiotherapy. Consider an orthopaedic referral if the patient is handicapped by deformities.
- Paroxysmal pain can be a problem in neuritis. Consider the use of carbamazepine or phenytoin.
- Constipation can be helped by ensuring an adequate fluid intake, bulking agents, suppositories or enemas.

- Obesity can be a problem for any patient with prolonged immobility. Consider referral to a dietician.
- Urinary problems are common in multiple sclerosis. Antibiotics for urinary tract infections may be needed. Try anticholinergics for bladder instability, e.g. oxybutynin 5 mg t.d.s. An opinion from a urology specialist may be needed. Catheterisation is occasionally required, and can be via a condom (Convene) or by intermittent self-catheterisation.
- Sexual dysfunction is common in multiple sclerosis. Consider sildenafil, or referral for counselling or a urology opinion.
- The Driver and Vehicle Licensing Agency should be informed by the patient. A disabled parking permit should be applied for.
- Depression is almost inevitable at some point in the life of every patient with multiple sclerosis (see p. 294). Stress in the carer is also common and is often overlooked.

HEAD INJURY

Patients with mild head injuries present commonly to GPs, often out of hours, and usually, initially, over the telephone. The decisions of whether to visit and whether to refer to A&E depend on the risk of the missed skull fracture.

Features requiring assessment

History • Motor vehicle accident • fall from a height • striking head on hard surface, e.g. concrete • striking side of head (temple) • loss of consciousness (>5 minutes) • retrograde amnesia • severe headache • drunk.

Examination Look for: • Altered consciousness level • focal neurological signs • bruising/haematoma, including around eyes and ears • blood/CSF from ears or nose • drunk • bulging fontanelle • irritable.

Management
- For analgesia use paracetamol, ibuprofen or codeine phosphate.
- If the patient is not visited or admitted, give standard head injury advice to contact the doctor if the following develop over the next 24 hours:
  – severe headache
  – vomiting
  – drowsiness
  – confusion.
- If any of the above symptoms do develop within 24 hours of a head injury the patient should be seen in an A&E department.

- Head injury in the elderly may present several days or weeks later, with symptoms and signs of a subdural haemorrhage: confusion, falls, loss of balance, memory loss. Obtain an urgent neurology opinion.

**Head injury under 1 year of age = ?Non-accidental injury.
Drunk with head injury = skull fracture until proven otherwise.**

PSYCHIATRY

DEPRESSION

Depression is the most common psychiatric problem of general practice.
There are well over 4000 suicides in the UK each year.

Diagnosis

History Ask about: ● low self-esteem ● low mood ● anhedonia ● poor
concentration ● thought of suicide ● poor sleep and appetite ● loss of libido ●
guilt ● irritability ● weight change.

Examination Look for: ● tearfulness ● slowed thinking and speech ●
indecisiveness ● sighing ● anxiety.

In children behavioural problems, school refusal and phobias may
represent depression, and in the elderly, complaining, confusion and
forgetfulness may be signs of depression.

When to suspect depression
Have a high index of suspicion of depression in the following: ● major illness
● chronic illness ● major life event (e.g. bereavement, unemployment, marital
breakdown) ● previous mental illness ● alcohol or drug abuse ● frequent
attendances ● carers.

Management
● Assess the risk of suicide (see p. 300).
● Explain the diagnosis to the patient:
  – depression is an illness
  – one might liken it to a deficiency state of chemical in the brain
  – the prognosis is excellent.

Non-drug treatment
● Continued GP support (offer follow-up with the same doctor).
● Family and friends, self-help groups.
● Counselling (e.g. with marital problems).
● Pyschologist (e.g. for cognitive behaviourial therapy).
● Community psychiatric nurse.

Prescribing
● Negotiate the use of drugs with the patient:
  – antidepressants are not addictive
  – they correct the chemical imbalance that is causing the patient's
    symptoms.

- Prescribe amitriptyline (if sedation is required for poor sleep) or imipramine (if sedation is not required). For both:
  - Start with 25 mg nocte for 4 nights, and increase by 25 mg a night every 4 nights.
  - Prescribe small quantities (dangerous in overdose).
  - Target range 150–200 mg daily.
  - Stop increasing the dose if side-effects become troublesome.
  - Use 50% of the normal dose in the elderly.
  - Side-effects: dry mouth, blurred vision, constipation, urinary retention, palpitations, weight gain, postural hypotension (in the elderly).
  - Contraindications: avoid in patients with recent heart attack, heart block, severe liver disease, mania.
- More commonly, though more expensive, selective serotonin reuptake inhibitors (SSRIs), e.g. fluoxetine (20 mg o.d.), paroxetine (20 mg o.d.) or citalopram (20 mg o.d.) are prescribed. SSRIs are particularly useful for young patients who may be intolerant of tricyclic side-effects, if there is a high risk of overdose or if a rapid onset of action is required.
  - Warn the patient that the therapeutic benefit will not be felt for the first 7–10 days.
  - Side-effects: common side-effects which usually settle within the first 2 weeks include nausea, nervousness and insomnia.
  - Contraindications: avoid if the patient enters a manic phase.
- If response is poor, consider third line antidepressants, e.g. venlafaxine, trazodone.
- Duration of treatment with antidepressants: 3–9 months. After the patient is feeling well, continue treatment for 3 or 4 months. Treatment should not be discontinued if the patient is approaching an emotionally challenging time. Abrupt withdrawal of SSRIs should be avoided by reducing the dose to one tablet or capsule on alternate days for 1 month before stopping completely.

Referral Referral to a psychiatrist is indicated with:
- uncertain diagnosis
- poor response to treatment at adequate doses
- suicide risk (immediate admission, see below)
- psychotic features
- behaviour disturbance, e.g. psychomotor retardation.

Special cases
- Postnatal depression (see p. 33).
- Manic depression: this is recognised by depressive episodes alternating with prolonged periods of euphoria. These are characterised by pressured speech, delusions of grandeur and loss of social inhibitions. Refer if the diagnosis is suspected. Admit if the patient is in danger.
- Bereavement (see p. 333).

ANXIETY

True anxiety neurosis interferes with the patient's normal daily activities. Milder forms of anxiety are extremely common, may accompany physical illness and can cause a variety of symptoms.

Diagnosis

History Patients most likely to suffer from anxiety are those with depression, stress, a major life event, somatisation symptoms, avoidance behaviour and dementia, and those who are frequent attenders.

Anxiety is a common cause of some typical complaints: • tiredness • headache • low back pain • dizziness • dysmenorrhoea.

Thyrotoxicosis can present with anxiety. It is often accompanied by weight loss, agitation and tremor.

Panic attacks involve the patient in a vicious circle of self-sustaining physical symptoms caused by anxiety.

In phobias the anxiety state is generated by a specific trigger.

Management

- Exclude physical disease at the initial consultation. Thereafter avoid overinvestigating, as this reinforces anxiety rather than relieving it.
- Treat any underlying depression (see p. 294).
- Symptomatic hyperventilation may be relieved by rebreathing expired air via a paper bag.

Non-drug treatment For chronic anxiety neurosis the treatment is mainly psychotherapeutic:

- Explain the condition to the patient.
- Reassure about the absence of physical disease.
- Explain symptoms in terms of autonomic stimulation.
- Try relaxation techniques: tapes, groups, yoga, swimming.
- Encourage regular exercise.
- Offer counselling.
- Self-help leaflets.
- Discuss complementary therapies.
- Offer cognitive behavioural therapy by referral to a psychologist, if available.

- Involve the psychiatric services if the patient's life is affected to any significant degree:
  - psychiatric social worker
  - community psychiatric nurse
  - consultant referral.

Prescribing

- For the acute, short-term relief of severe anxiety, e.g. in panic attacks, use diazepam 2–5 mg tablets t.d.s., as required. The maximum duration of treatment should be 14 days. Alternatively, prescribe propranolol 10–40 mg t.d.s., as required.
- For chronic anxiety consider an SSRI, e.g. paroxetine 20 mg o.d., or a tricyclic, e.g. clomipramine 10–75 mg o.d.
- For chronic agitation, e.g. in dementia, chlorpromazine 25–50 mg nocte is more appropriate.

OBSESSIVE–COMPULSIVE DISORDER

Obsessive–compulsive disorder (OCD) is a neurobiological condition which causes the patient to feel compelled repeatedly to think, speak or act-out irrational rituals, such as hand washing, touching objects or chanting mantras. The spectrum of severity is wide, with the mildest form almost going unnoticed by the patient and family, e.g. the need for a child to organise their teddy bears or dolls in a certain way. The most severe cases are disablingly time-consuming and can provoke extreme anxiety.

- OCD affects about 1% of children and adolescents.
- It tends to run in families.
- Children often keep their symptoms a secret.

Diagnosis

History Ask about:

- unwanted thoughts or ideas that keep coming into the mind
- the need to perform rituals
- anxiety at the thought of not completing the rituals
- how long it takes to perform the ritual each time
- how many times a day the ritual has to be repeated
- interference with daily life, schoolwork, sleep
- other mental illness, e.g. brain injury, tics, Tourette syndrome.

Management

In mild cases the patient and family need reassurance that the condition is usually self-limiting.

Referral

- Patients who are upset by the OCD.
- Patients who take more than an hour a day to perform their rituals.
- Patients in whom the rituals interfere with everyday life.

Treatment

The SSRI group of antidepressants are the most useful for the drug treatment of OCD (e.g. fluoxetine 20–60 mg o.d.). The other effective treatment for OCD is cognitive behavioural therapy. A combination of the two is usually offered by psychiatrists.

INSOMNIA

Insomnia can be divided into acute and chronic. The chronic variety is more common in the elderly.

Diagnosis

History Take a careful history and try to decide if the problem is long-term or of recent onset.

The causes of acute insomnia include: • trauma, physical or psychological • jet lag • change of environment, e.g. admission to a nursing home.

The causes of chronic insomnia include: • day-time sleeping, e.g. in the elderly • stimulants, e.g. caffeine • drugs, e.g. SSRIs • physical symptoms, e.g. pain, cough, nasal obstruction • anxiety/depression (see pp. 294 and 296).

Explore patients' expectations: are they looking for a cure or short-term relief?

Management

- Explain that insomnia is not a disease.
- Treat the underlying cause, if any (see above).
- Try to avoid prescribing for chronic insomnia.
- Offer self-help leaflet.
- Advise a regular bedtime routine.
- Advise avoidance of stimulants, e.g. caffeine, alcohol.
- Are the patient's expectations unrealistic?
- For short-term treatment requiring rapid relief of symptoms, i.e. no longer than 2 weeks, prescribe, e.g.:
  - temazepam 10–20 mg nocte, *or*
  - zopiclone 7.5–15 mg nocte.

> **Addiction to benzodiazepines**
> Explain the addiction potential of benzodiazepines to the patient and record in the notes that this has been discussed. A number of successful litigation cases against doctors over the prescribing of benzodiazepines have hinged on the fact that the patients were not informed of the addiction potential of these drugs. State the maximum safe duration of treatment (2 weeks) to the patient and explain that drugs are not a long-term cure.

PSYCHOSOMATIC ILLNESS

Patients with psychosomatic illnesses all share the belief that they are physically unwell. The frequent attender, chronic somatiser and heartsink patient may all come under this heading.

 Negative emotions in the doctor are common with this group of patients. Recognising this is an important step in coping.

Diagnosis

History Psychosomatic illnesses may be difficult to distinguish from organic disease initially. The patient with globus hystericus, for example, may present with a straightforward sore throat.

However, a number of suspicious features make the possibility of a psychosomatic illness increasingly likely: multiple, unconnected physical symptoms; 'vague' symptoms such as spasms, churning or pressure; impossible symptoms, such as pain all over; and symptoms that defy treatment, such as wind, bloating and electric shocks.

Examination Satisfy yourself that the physical symptoms have been adequately explored by examination, investigation and referral, if indicated.

Management

- Gently, but firmly, inform patients that their symptoms, while real, are not due to physical disease. Many patients are difficult to reassure, but an unwavering message is important. The slightest doubt in the doctor's mind is soon picked up by patients and used to reinforce their neurosis.
- Many patients will have emotional, social or family problems. Some may be clinically depressed (see p. 294). Some patients may have a justifiable phobia, e.g. after losing a close friend to cancer. Attempt to explore these areas.

- Encourage the patient to expect less of the doctor's abilities to cure the physical symptoms.
- Encourage the patient to lead a normal life despite the symptoms, rather than be dominated by them.

The above process is often spread over many consultations and may be repeated as patients 'relapse'.

Referral Referral to a specialist to exclude organic disease can be a useful way of reassuring patients that they are not physically unwell.

Referral to a psychiatrist is sometimes necessary to lighten the load on the GP. Some psychiatrists have an interest in hypochondriasis. The community psychiatric nurse or social worker can help explore emotional, social and family problems. The clinical psychologist may be able to provide the patient with training in behavioural methods of coping with physical and mental symptoms.

FATIGUE

Fatigue is a common presenting symptom in general practice. It is often described as: tired all the time, exhausted, lacking energy, sleepy, worn out.

Depression or anxiety are probably the commonest causes. Exclude physical causes at the initial consultation.

Physical causes of fatigue:

- acute infection (e.g. flu-like illness)
- postviral
- alcohol abuse
- heart failure
- malignancy (e.g. lung, breast, bowel, lymphoma)
- diabetes
- hypothyroidism
- degenerative neurological disease (usually described as weakness)
- chronic infection (e.g. TB, bronchiectasis)
- anaemia.

Diagnosis

Physical causes should be excluded largely on the history, supported by examination of the relevant system(s).

Investigations should be directed towards suspected physical illnesses, although normal FBC, ESR and TFTs help to reassure both patient and doctor.

It is useful to ask yourself:

- Why is the patient consulting?
- Have I excluded disease?
- Is there a hidden agenda (e.g. marital problems)?
- What are the expectations of cure?
- Does the patient have a dependent personality?

Chronic fatigue syndrome This is characterised by a history of fatigue lasting 6 months or more, accompanied by widespread muscle pains and profound weakness. Investigations fail to reveal a physical cause. The condition lasts from a few months to several years. Depression may coexist with chronic fatigue.

Management

- If the history suggests depression, explore and treat (see p. 294).
- Explain to the patient that you have been unable to find a physical cause. Acknowledge the patient's problem of fatigue.
- If family or social problems emerge, it may be helpful to pursue these if time allows. Alternatively, offer another appointment.
- It may be necessary to correct the patient's expectations of the doctor, e.g. 'I need a tonic, Doctor'.
- Chronic fatigue is best managed with empathy and encouragement. The ME Association (see p. 386) is a valuable source of support. Medical certificates should be issued to the patient who claims to be too fatigued to work. The Benefits Agency generally takes a sympathetic view of this condition.

Referral Referral is indicated if:

- a physical disease is suggested but cannot be ruled out (e.g. a suspicion of bowel cancer)
- depression proves difficult to treat (see p. 294)
- help is needed with psychosocial problems (e.g. family therapy)
- anxiety cannot be treated successfully in general practice.

SUICIDE

There are over 4000 deaths per year in the UK due to suicide. The majority of victims have consulted a GP prior to death.

> Most suicide patients suffer from a mental illness: • depression (most common) • alcoholism • schizophrenia.

Premorbid diagnosis

History A number of factors in the history are associated with a higher risk of suicide: • increasing age • male sex • divorced/separated/living alone • psychiatric illness • alcoholism • economic stress • family history of alcoholism/mental illness/suicide.

Among women, suicide has also been associated with: • loss of mother by death or separation before age 12 • three or more children under 3 years old • lack of job/close relationship.

Also ask about: • preoccupation with suicide • active plans made for suicide • fear of irresistible urge to commit suicide • delusions of persecution • auditory hallucinations instructing suicide.

Management

- Consider the possibility of suicide when dealing with mental illness.
- An open discussion with the patient of the risk of suicide is very useful, e.g. 'Do you ever think life is not worth going on with?' Most suicidal patients are grateful for this.
- Consider risk factors (see above).
- Try to establish the level of risk.
- Try to achieve a psychiatric diagnosis in simple terms: depression, psychosis, alcoholism, etc.
- Treat the underlying disorder:
  - depression (see p. 294)
  - alcoholism (see p. 311)
  - psychosis (see p. 305).
- Avoid overprescribing large quantities of drugs when seeing patients in a depressed state. Drug overdose with recently dispensed antidepressants is common.
- Consider admission to hospital:
  - via A&E if the patient has taken a drug overdose
  - via a psychiatric unit, by voluntary or compulsory admission (see p. 309).
- Frequent follow-up of depressed or disturbed patients enables smaller quantities of drugs to be dispensed, is good clinical practice, and enables the GP more accurately to assess a rising suicide risk.

EATING DISORDERS

ANOREXIA NERVOSA

Anorexia nervosa is most common in upper social class women, between the ages of 15 and 25. It affects up to 2% in this group. The mortality is 5–10%.

Diagnosis

History Ask about: • progressive weight loss • reduction in food intake • distorted body image • morbid fear of getting fat • indifference to food intake.

In other causes of weight loss, such as malignancy, thyrotoxicosis and malabsorption, patients usually acknowledge they are losing weight.

The patient with anorexia nervosa is at increased risk of: • confusional states • depression • suicide • electrolyte imbalance • dehydration • fitting • death (5–10%) • amenorrhoea.

Ordinary dieting can easily be distinguished from anorexia nervosa by a normal response to food in the former, e.g. a craving for high-calorie foods.

Management

Admit the patient to hospital if:

- **severe depression is present (see p. 294)**
- **weight loss has been rapid and persistent**
- **the weight is below 60% of normal for sex and height.**

Compulsory admission may be necessary (see p. 307).

Ask about emotional difficulties with e.g. parents, peers, boyfriend. Discuss aspects of adolescence such as sexual maturation, leaving home, adult responsibilities.

Frequent follow-up is important if the patient is to be managed in general practice. Consultations should include weight, BP and pulse, food intake and attitudes to food and weight gain. If amenorrhoea is prolonged, consider arranging bone densitometry (increased risk of osteoporosis). Less severe cases commonly resolve with time, encouragement and support. Consider referral to a pyschiatric department or specialist eating disorder unit (if available).

BULIMIA NERVOSA

Bulimia nervosa is characterised by avoidance of calorie intake by vomiting or purgation after overeating in binges. It is difficult to diagnose as the weight is often normal and the behaviour secretive. Half of patients with bulimia have previously suffered anorexia nervosa.

Management

Management is as for anorexia nervosa (see p. 303).

DEMENTIA

About 5% of people over 65 have moderate to severe dementia. The majority of cases are due to Alzheimer's-type or multi-infarct dementia. The frequency increases with age.

Seventy-five per cent of patients with Alzheimer's disease die within 2–4 years of diagnosis.

Diagnosis

History Dementia is characterised by slowly progressive deterioration in cognitive function: • memory difficulties (particularly short-term) • speech difficulties • personality changes • uncharacteristic behaviour • loss of abstract reasoning.

These are often noticed first by a relative or neighbour.

There should be no change in consciousness level.

Examination The abbreviated mental test is helpful:

1. Age.
2. Time.
3. Remember address: '42 West Street'.
4. Year.
5. 'Where are we now?'
6. 'Do you know who I am?'
7. Date of birth.
8. Year of First World War.
9. Name of present Prime Minister.
10. Count backwards from 20 to 1.

A score of less than 8 is abnormal.

To exclude secondary causes look for: • depression • Parkinson's syndrome • hypothyroidism • deafness • stigmata of alcoholism • acute steroid withdrawal.

Neurological examination should be normal. Focal signs prompt urgent referral.

Investigations (dementia screen) • FBC and ESR • U&E, LFTs and glucose • TFT • vitamin B_{12} and folate • VDRL (or equivalent).

Management

All new cases should be referred to a neurologist if the diagnosis is uncertain or unusual (for a CT brain), or to a psychogeriatrician, if available. The patient should be accompanied by a relative.

Long-term problems

- Depression: treat in the usual way (see p. 294).
- Aggression (see below).
- Loss of driving licence: advise patient/relative to inform the Driver and Vehicle Licensing Agency.
- Wandering and other safety aspects: Medic Alert bracelet.
- Financial difficulties: suggest early application for enduring power of attorney (see a solicitor).

Prescribing Treatment with major tranquillisers reduces the risk of self-harm:

- Agitation at night: e.g. promazine (Sparine) 25–75 mg o.n.
- Aggression: e.g. Risperidone 1 mg o.d. or b.d.
- Nocturnal wakefulness: haloperidol 2 mg b.d.
- Depression: (see p. 294).
- Sexual disinhibition: benperidol 0.25 mg o.d. to 0.5 mg t.d.s.

Use the lowest dose possible to achieve the desired effect.

Side-effects Extrapyramidal effects and postural hypotension.

Support • Community psychiatric nurse • district nurse • incontinence advisor • Social Services and benefits • day centre • respite admission • residential/nursing-home care • Alzheimer's Society (see p. 384).

DISTURBED BEHAVIOUR

The GP may be called to attend a patient whose behaviour or speech is abnormal and characterised by delusions, hallucinations or acute confusion.
This behaviour may have:

- Functional causes: e.g. schizophrenia, mania, depressive psychosis.
- Organic causes: e.g. hypoglycaemia, head injury, brain tumour, encephalitis, drug side-effects, septicaemia, alcoholism.

Management

> ⚠️ **The first priority is to gain control of the situation. The patient may already be calm and willing to try and answer questions, but some patients may be aggressive or give the impression of being frightened and ready to strike out at the doctor. (For violent behaviour, see below.)**

Sedation If sedation is necessary to gain control, the patient should be given haloperidol 10 mg i.m. The dose may be repeated up to three times if necessary.

Gain as much information as possible about the patient from a relative, the notes, other partners, the community psychiatric nurse or receptionist, and obtain details of current medication.

Admission to hospital? Consider admission if the patient's behaviour is dangerous to himself/herself or others, or there is serious physical illness or an undiagnosed acute mental disorder.

The patient may not need admitting if there has been a gradual deterioration in mental function (e.g. dementia), or there is a minor physical illness (e.g. delirium due to fever of tonsillitis).

Medical or psychiatric admission? A patient with an acute psychiatric emergency should look generally well physically. There should be no suggestion of an acute medical problem and the predominant features of the illness should be a disturbance of thought or behaviour.

If the patient is unwilling to go into hospital, consider compulsory admission (p. 307).

Disturbed behaviour after psychiatric discharge from hospital may remain within socially acceptable limits. The community psychiatric nurse should review the patient regularly. Acute worsening of the patient's condition will probably warrant readmission.

VIOLENCE

Violence against doctors is increasing. It can be verbal as well as physical. Some violence is due to organic disease, such as hypoglycaemia and cerebral events. Some patients are simply violent people.

Some hints for preventing violence

- Have a written procedure for dealing with complaints.

- Listen sympathetically. Do not get defensive.
- Avoid physical confrontation. Talk to the person firmly but calmly, and do not provoke them.

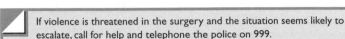

> If violence is threatened in the surgery and the situation seems likely to escalate, call for help and telephone the police on **999**.
>
> If violence appears likely while on a visit, leave immediately. Call the person by telephone and tell him or her you will only return to the house with a police escort.

After an episode of threatened or actual violence
- Record the details of the episode accurately in the notes.
- Discuss the events with your partners. Similar episodes with the same patient may be revealed.
- Removing a person from the practice's list is the only way of guaranteeing safety for doctors and staff in the future. Inform the Health Authority of your decision; they will contact the patient.
- Before removing a patient from the list, ensure there are no reasonable grounds to suspect an underlying illness to account for his or her behaviour.
- If a complaint was involved, inform your defence organisation.
- Consider criminal proceedings in cases of assault.

SECTIONING

The compulsory admission of a patient to hospital is most often used for suicide risk and acute psychosis. It allows the GP to admit a person, against his or her will, to a psychiatric unit under the Mental Health Act 1983.

Before seeing the patient
- Prior knowledge of the patient is useful. Obtain the GP records.
- Consider your own safety. Call the police if in doubt. See violence, page 306.
- The patient may need sedating. Check you have a major tranquilliser, e.g. haloperidol 30 mg i.m.

Requirements of the act
- The patient must be suffering from a mental illness, e.g. depression or psychosis, and not just be antisocial, drunk, etc.
- Admission is in the interest of the patient's health or safety or to protect others, e.g. if there is a high risk of suicide or the patient is dangerous.
- Voluntary admission is preferred if possible.

How to organise a compulsory admission

- Telephone the duty psychiatrist to discuss the case and request formal admission.
- A psychiatrist, an approved social worker (ASW) and a doctor who knows the patient (usually the GP) each need to assess the patient in order to admit under Section 2 (28-day compulsory admission for assessment and treatment). Arrangements are usually coordinated by the ASW.
- On the patient's discharge from hospital, ensure that a suitable follow-up plan is in place.

Mental Health Act 1983

Section 2: Admission for assessment and treatment up to 28 days.

Section 3: Admission for treatment for up to 6 months initially.

Section 4: Emergency admission for up to 72 hours.

Section 136: Removal from a public place to a place of safety by the police.

Administration

Submit a local authority claim form for payment, as arranging compulsory admission attracts a fee. Remember to state your mileage.

BENZODIAZEPINE ADDICTION

Many patients in general practice, especially the elderly, may have been on long-term repeat prescriptions for benzodiazepines.

Management

Patients who want to stop taking benzodiazepines

- Offer continuing support, including the prescribing of drugs if necessary.
- Explain the effect of benzodiazepines on memory and judgement and the effects of tolerance and dependence.
- Change to a short-acting drug, such as diazepam or temazepam, if the patient is not already taking one.
- Agree with the patient the timetable for withdrawal. This may need to be as slow as a quarter of a tablet a month.
- Address the psychiatric needs of the patient, e.g. depression (see p. 294), anxiety (see p. 296).
- Allow the patient to keep a small supply of tablets in the house, 'in case of emergency'.
- Suggest counselling or self-help groups.

Patients who do not want to stop
- A patient's commitment to stopping may fluctuate.
- Explain the risks as above and record the discussion in the notes. (Recent cases of litigation have made this more important.)
- Offer help with psychiatric problems.
- Try at a future date to encourage patients to stop, e.g. by including with their repeat prescription an invitation to discuss the issue with the doctor.

OPIATE ADDICTION

There are two new cases of opiate addiction per GP per year in the UK on average. The trend is increasing and there are higher rates in city practices. Opiate addiction is associated with a 20-fold excess mortality for age.

Diagnosis

History Opiate addiction presents in a variety of ways to the GP, but most commonly:

- The patient admits to drug abuse and wants help.

> Some addicts present with withdrawal symptoms in an attempt to gain a prescription for opiates or benzodiazepines. It is wise to resist, especially if they are not known to the GP and if this is the first consultation.

- The patient wants a prescription to prevent or treat withdrawal symptoms.
- Drug abuse complicates or leads to other medical conditions: pain, hepatitis, HIV, depression and suicide, sepsis, overdose.

Take a history of drug use to distinguish between the intermittent drug misuser and the physically dependent addict. Validate the history, as necessary, by telephoning the patient's usual GP and consultant psychiatrist.

Examination Examine for evidence of injection, hepatitis, sepsis.

Investigations
- Urine sample for drug screen.
- Blood tests, for hepatitis B and C and HIV status.

Management
- Deal with any urgent medical problems not requiring a prescription for opiates or other psychotropic medication, e.g. sepsis.

- Offer a longer consultation within the next 2–3 days, to provide a more thorough evaluation of the problem, before deciding on long-term management.
- Patients requesting opiates may become aggressive if refused. The management of the aggressive patient is dealt with on page 306.
- Counsel for HIV testing if appropriate (see p. 192). Offer hepatitis B immunisation (see p. 201).
- The occasional drug misuser may only need advice, support and referral to the local drug counselling service or self-help groups.
- Patients with a short history of drug abuse may require the above, but with prescriptions and advice on the treatment of withdrawal symptoms: Imodium for diarrhoea, clonidine for sweating and propranolol for anxiety.

Advice
- Offer continuing medical support for general health matters.
- Advise about not sharing needles, safe injection techniques and needle-exchange programmes.
- Advocate smoking rather than injecting.

> For the established opiate addict a withdrawal programme should be devised, based on the gradual reduction of methadone. This should be provided by the local specialist in drug addiction, who determines the prescribing and follow-up schedule for the patient. Writing out the prescriptions can be shared with the GP.

Prescribing controlled drugs (For the main rules, see p. 325.)
Additional rules for addicts include:

- There should be a written contract from the specialist outlining the duration of treatment and rate of withdrawal. No extra drugs should be given. Lost drugs are the patient's responsibility. The commonest drug used for controlled withdrawal is methadone.
- Discuss with the pharmacist or dispenser. Daily dispensing of the daily ration helps prevent the patient taking it all at once or from selling it. The prescription should be marked 'supervised consumption'. This ensures that the patient has to consume each daily ration in front of the pharmacist and should be continued for the first 3 months of treatment or until compliance is assured. It is easier to use a blue FP10 (GP10 in Scotland), as there is space for the pharmacist to record up to 14 daily doses dispensed. Dispense 2-days' supply on Saturday if the chemist closes on the Sunday.
- Write 'Methadone mixture 1 mg/ml' on the prescription.
- Inform other GPs in the practice. Aim for care by one GP.
- Ongoing support from the drug counsellor is vital.

Dealing with drug abusers can be very difficult and specialist help should be sought early in most cases. As with tobacco and alcohol abuse, relapse is common.

ALCOHOL ABUSE

Alcohol abuse affects women as well as men, the elderly as well as the young, and all social classes. On a national basis the average GP will probably have 5–10 alcoholic patients per 2000 population per year.

High-risk groups include: • publicans • caterers • members of the armed forces • business executives.

Diagnosis
Alcohol abuse presents in a number of ways:

- a complaint from a relative or friend
- a request from the patient for help with drinking
- memory loss
- stress
- poor performance
- fatigue
- depression
- gastritis
- an incidental finding.

History The first task is to establish a diagnosis of alcohol abuse. Ask about:
- The level of alcohol consumption. Answers from patients are notoriously understated and should be confirmed with the patient's partner if possible.
- Memory gaps or amnesia.
- Any preoccupation with alcohol.
- Guilt about drinking.
- A feeling they should cut down.
- Annoyance about criticism of drinking habit.
- Needing a drink early in the day to feel normal.

Examination If appropriate, look for: • hypertension • obesity/malnourishment • jaundice • hepatomegaly • cardiomegaly • arrhythmias • encephalopathy (tremor) • polyneuropathy.

Investigations Investigations are not always necessary. However, the following are useful:

- FBC for the macrocytosis of chronic alcohol excess
- γ-GT, to challenge a patient's denial of drinking

- LFTs
- urine to screen for other drugs.

Management

 The management of alcohol abuse is a lengthy and time-consuming business and can be spread over more than one consultation.

Crisis intervention Occasionally the patient presents with an acute medical or psychiatric problem due to alcohol abuse:

- Severe depression: there is a high risk of suicide in this group of patients. Admit to a psychiatric unit, by compulsory admission if necessary (see p. 307).
- Acute withdrawal complications, such as fitting, atrial fibrillation and delirium tremens: admit under the medical team.
- Acute complications of chronic alcohol abuse: these include pancreatitis, hepatitis, bleeding oesophageal varices and encephalopathy. Admit under the medical team.

Planned intervention

As alcoholism is not considered to be a psychiatric disease by itself, any treatment given must be with the consent of the patient. Often the cry for help comes from the spouse, in which case try to support the spouse also.

Detoxification
- Establish the patient's motivation to detoxify.
- Underline to patients that they are responsible for their drinking and for the success of the detoxification.
- Refer for inpatient detoxification if any of the following apply:
  – history of withdrawal fits or delirium tremens
  – there are coexisting medical problems
  – any psychiatric condition
  – inadequate domestic support
  – misuser of other drugs.

Home detoxification regimen Prescribe:
- chlordiazepoxide (Librium) orally 5 mg and 10 mg tablets:
  – 20 mg q.d.s. for 1 day
  – 20 mg t.d.s. for 1 day

- 15 mg t.d.s. for 1 day
- 10 mg t.d.s. for 1 day
- 10 mg b.d. for 1 day
- 5 mg b.d. for 1 day
- vitamin B complex 1 tablet daily
- vitamin C tablet 1 daily.

Ask the pharmacist to dispense the drugs on a daily basis if the patient is likely to comply poorly with medication or become dependent on benzodiazepines.

> Help and advice from the District Drug and Alcohol Team is useful, if it is available.

Long-term management
- Reiterate to patients that the responsibility for drinking is theirs.
- Encourage contact with self-help groups:
  - Alcoholics Anonymous (see p. 384)
  - Al-Anon Family Groups (for relatives) (see p. 384).
- Treat any contributory illness, such as depression (see p. 294).

SMOKING

Smoking is now recognised as an addiction treatable at the expense of the NHS.

Treatment should be offered to smokers who express a desire to quit, and should form part of an advice and encouragement programme.

NRT (nicotine-replacement therapy) and Bupropion are the two forms of treatment available on the NHS.

Formulations
- Nicotine skin-patches, gum, lozenges, sublingual tablets, inhalators or nasal spray.
- Bupropion tablets. Generally, patients should be prescribed Bupropion only after unsuccessful attempts at quitting with NRT.

Contraindications
- Age under 18 years.
- Pregnancy and breast-feeding.
- Unstable cardiovascular disease.

NRT patch

Choosing a patch There are currently three brands of patch and all come in three strengths. Smokers of over 20 cigarettes a day need the strongest patch to start with; smokers of 10 cigarettes or less a day can start with the medium-strength patch. Smokers who start smoking first thing in the morning need a 24-hour patch (e.g. Nicotinell or NiQuitin); later starters can use a 16-hour patch (Nicorette).

Using the patches Prescribe 2 weeks supply on an NHS prescription and get the patient to set a quit date. The patient stops smoking on the quit date and uses one patch every day. If they are still abstinent after 2 weeks then a further prescription for 2 weeks can be issued under the NHS. Further patches must be purchased by the patient. Each brand of patch has its own schedule for dose reduction and total duration of use.

Bupropion

Bupropion is prescribed on the NHS for 4 weeks initially and a further 4 weeks if abstinence is maintained. The patient's quit date is set for 2 weeks after the medication is started. The starting dose is 150 mg o.d., increased to 150 mg b.d. after the first 6 days. If there are risk factors for seizure the dose should be kept at 150 mg o.d. throughout.

Further attempts at quitting should not be funded by the NHS within 6 months.

Each practice should have access to a lead person on smoking who can offer support to patients attempting to quit. Practice nurses and health visitors are valuable resources in this role.

HAEMATOLOGY

ANAEMIA

Patients with anaemia are diagnosed either because they look anaemic, have the symptoms of anaemia or are found incidentally to be anaemic.

Diagnosis

History Ask about:

- Bleeding: heavy periods are a common cause of iron-deficiency anaemia. Rectal bleeding is the other common cause.
- Diet: the elderly often take a diet low in iron. Vegetarians are also at risk.
- A past history of iron-deficiency anaemia, which raises the chance of another episode of the same.
- Symptoms of anaemia: tiredness, breathlessness, exhaustion and palpitations can all be caused by anaemia. Angina can be unmasked or exacerbated by becoming anaemic.
- Symptoms occasionally accompanying anaemias: bruising and infections suggest aplastic anaemia. Paraesthesia of the feet can occur in pernicious anaemia. Chronic disease can cause anaemia, e.g. renal failure, inflammatory bowel disease and rheumatoid arthritis. Cancer often causes anaemia.

Examination In general practice there is usually little to add by examining the asymptomatic patient other than to look at the conjunctivae for pallor. The yellowish appearance of the face in pernicious anaemia is characteristic.

Investigations

- Full blood count: the first test is the FBC and film. This alone is sufficient to confirm the presence of anaemia, which is characterised by a Hb less than:
  - 12.5 g/dl for men
  - 11.5 g/dl for women.

Macrocytosis

If there is a macrocytosis on the FBC (mean cell volume >96 fl) this can be due to:

- Hypothyroidism. (Check TSH.)
- Alcoholism. (Take alcohol history or check γ-GT.)
- Vitamin B_{12} or folate deficiency. (Check blood levels.)
- Pregnancy.
- Rarely:
  - malignancy (check ESR)
  - radiotherapy
  - liver disease (check LFTs).

- Iron-deficiency anaemia is characterised by a low mean cell volume (<76 fl) and a low mean cell Hb concentration (<30 g/dl), and should be confirmed by checking for a low serum iron (<15 µmol/l in men; 14 µmol/l in women).
- Total iron binding capacity: a high total iron binding capacity (>70 µmol/l in men; 74 µmol/l in women) supports the diagnosis of iron-deficiency anaemia. A low total iron binding capacity (<45 in men, <40 in women) suggests the anaemia of chronic disease.

Management

Iron-deficiency anaemia

 Where there is no obvious cause for the anaemia (e.g. heavy periods), the patient should be referred for investigation of the gastrointestinal tract. Occult malignancy occasionally comes to light after presenting with anaemia.

Mild anaemia (Hb >7 g/dl) can be treated with ferrous sulphate tablets 200 mg daily, rechecking the full blood count after 1 month. Attention should be given to the underlying cause, i.e. dietary advice or treatment of menorrhagia.

Some patients cannot tolerate ferrous sulphate tablets due to gastrointestinal side-effects. Try ferrous fumarate in these cases. If oral iron fails to correct the anaemia, or if tablets cannot be tolerated, use iron sorbitol injection. (See *Data Sheet Compendium*, published by Datapharm, 12 Whitehall, London SW1A 2DY for dose schedule.)

 Patients with severe anaemia (Hb <7 g/dl) who are symptomatic should be considered for blood transfusion in hospital.

Anaemia of chronic disease Many chronic diseases are accompanied by a mild anaemia with an Hb of around 10 g/dl. These patients are usually asymptomatic from the anaemia and require no treatment as such. In fact, their anaemia is often refractory to treatment.

Macrocytic anaemia Treatment is of the underlying cause, as identified above.

Vitamin B_{12} deficiency is usually due to pernicious anaemia, malabsorption of B_{12} from the gut (due to e.g. inflammatory bowel disease) or dietary deficiency. Check with a blood test for the presence of intrinsic factor antibodies. A positive result is strongly suggestive of pernicious anaemia.

Treat with intramuscular hydroxocobalamin 1 mg every 3 days for 2 weeks, then once every 3 months for life. Check an FBC after 1 month to make sure the macrocytosis has gone and to exclude iron-deficiency anaemia, which may complicate B_{12} treatment.

Folate deficiency is usually caused by malabsorption due to bowel disease, but rarely it is caused by dietary deficiency. Treatment is with oral folic acid 5 mg daily. Vitamin B_{12} deficiency should be excluded prior to commencing treatment with folic acid, as peripheral neuropathy in B_{12} deficiency can be precipitated by the administration of folate.

Anaemia of pregnancy See page 30.

Other causes of anaemia Other anaemias should be investigated and treated by referral to the haematology outpatient department.

HAEMOGLOBINOPATHIES

Screening
In general practice, patients with anaemia should be screened for thalassaemia and sickle cell traits if they are from Mediterranean, South-East Asian or Afro-Caribbean races.

Investigations
Blood should be sent for haemoglobin electrophoresis. Most results are normal, but mild abnormalities commonly demonstrate thalassaemia or sickle cell traits. These usually cause no more than a mild, asymptomatic anaemia and a slightly reduced mean cell volume and mean cell haemoglobin.

Counselling
Consider referral for genetic testing and counselling if the patient is contemplating starting a family. Refer to a department of clinical genetics.

Sickle cell disease
Homozygous sufferers should have specialist involvement from a haematology outpatient department.

Be alert for a sickle crisis:

- **sepsis**
- **painful swelling of the hands and feet**
- **rapid enlargement of the spleen**
- **acute fall in haemoglobin.**

If suspected, admit the patient.

SPLENECTOMY

Patients without a functioning spleen have a 12-fold increased risk of infection from *Pneumococcus*, *Haemophilus influenzae*, *Neisseria meningitidis* and malaria compared with people with a normal spleen.

Immunisation
Four vaccines should be given at the time of splenectomy or as soon as possible after surgery:

- pneumococcal vaccine (reimmunise every 5–10 years)
- Hib vaccine (single dose)
- meningococcal group C vaccine (single dose)
- influenza vaccine (reimmunise anually).

Antibiotics
To help prevent pneumococcal infection in asplenic patients, give penicillin V 500 mg o.d. Continue to the age of 16 years in children. For adults some authorities recommend treatment for 2 years post-splenectomy (period of greatest risk); others advise lifelong prophylaxis.

Have a low threshold for prescribing antibiotics for infections. (Prescribe 'standby' amoxycillin to start at once if necessary.)

Malaria
Explain the importance of taking antimalarials in view of the increased risk (see p. 185).

TERMINAL CARE

BREAKING BAD NEWS

Telling patients or their relatives about a terminal condition is never an easy job, but the GP, with a prior knowledge of the patient and family, is often the best person to break the bad news.

Before seeing the patient
Get all the facts beforehand, allow plenty of time and ensure there will be no interruptions.

Facts often needed include: ● prognosis ● symptoms to be expected ● treatment and side-effects.

What to say and how to say it
● Tell the truth.
● Recap on knowledge already gained, e.g. 'What did they tell you in hospital?'
● Stick to the terms used by the patient, e.g. 'growth', 'tumour'.
● Give factual knowledge in simple terms, with pauses for the patient to interrupt and ask questions.
● Allow the patient to be defensive.
● Do not give more information than the patient wants.
● Try to discover the patient's fears.
● Give positive aspects, e.g. professional support, effective analgesia.

Follow-up Make a further appointment to see the patient, who may feel isolated. Offer telephone access in the meantime. Suggest district nurse involvement.

The patient may come to terms with the realities of the illness only after several discussions along the above lines.

Administration
All patients with less than 6 months' life expectancy are eligible for Attendance Allowance, irrespective of their need for care. Apply with form DS1500 (available from Social Services). The reverse side of the form is for the GP to claim a fee for this service from the DSS.

PAIN

The thought of being in pain due to a terminal illness frightens many patients. This fear is sometimes not stated.

Pain and anxiety reinforce one another. Anxiolytics can help control pain. Ask patients if they have pain, rather than waiting for them to volunteer it.

Management of pain relief in palliative care

- Diagnose the cause of pain if possible, e.g. tumour mass, bone metastases, nerve compression, abdominal distension.
- Think of non-drug methods of pain relief, e.g. radiotherapy, surgery, relief of constipation, draining ascites, psychosocial support.
- Do not forget to treat anxiety as an adjunct to pain relief (see p. 296).
- Always bear in mind the potential side-effects of drugs (see constipation, p. 329, and vomiting, p. 326).

Using combinations of analgesics early, rather than increasing the dose of one drug, is often useful. The resulting effect is often greater than the sum of the individual drugs.

Examples of useful analgesics
(See controlled drugs, p. 325.)

Mild analgesics
- Paracetamol 500 mg, 1–2 tablets 4–6-hourly p.r.n.
- Ibuprofen 400 mg, 1 tablet p.r.n.

Moderate analgesics
- Co-proxamol, 1–2 tablets 4–6-hourly p.r.n.
- Dihydrocodeine 30 mg, 1–2 tablets 4–6-hourly p.r.n
- Diclofenac 75 mg b.d, 1 tablet.

Strong analgesics
- Morphine sulphate elixir 10 mg/5 ml.
- Morphine sulphate solution 20 mg/ml.
- Morphine sulphate Continus tablets (MST) 10, 15, 30, 60, 100 and 200 mg tablets.
- Morphine sulphate suppositories 10, 20 and 30 mg.
- Diamorphine injection 5, 10, 30, 100 and 500 mg.

How to achieve the correct dose of opiate
- Once it becomes apparent that mild and moderate analgesics are inadequate, substitute oral morphine 5 mg 4-hourly. Regular 4-hourly dosage is preferable, as the aim is total analgesia, without breakthrough pain.
- Increase the dose if necessary by titrating against the pain and giving more morphine, but at the same 4-hourly intervals.

Converting oral morphine solution to MST

- Once satisfactory pain control has been achieved, divide the total 24-hourly dose of morphine by 2 and give this dose as MST at 12-hour intervals, e.g. 10 ml of morphine sulphate elixir every 4 hours at 10 mg/5 ml equates to 60 mg b.d. of MST.
- As time goes on and the patient develops a tolerance to opiates, the dose of morphine will need to be increased. Use additional morphine sulphate elixir as a top-up initially, and when pain control is again achieved, divide the total 24-hourly dose by 2 and convert to the new dose of MST.
- Giving an NSAID such as diclofenac tablets 50 mg t.d.s. as well as the morphine can improve pain control, avoiding the side-effects of increased doses of opiates.

> Morphine sulphate suppositories are useful if a patient whose pain is well controlled on oral medication starts vomiting (unless the vomiting is due to too high a dose of morphine).

Converting oral morphine to diamorphine

- Diamorphine injections are useful for short-term relief of severe pain in e.g. MI. In terminal care, however, diamorphine can be given by subcutaneous infusion via a syringe driver. For practical purposes, injected diamorphine is about three times as powerful as oral morphine on a dose-for-dose basis. For example, the patient requiring MST 90 mg b.d. would need 60 mg diamorphine over 24 hours.
- Common side-effects of opiates include:
  - constipation
  - nausea and vomiting
  - drowsiness
  - anorexia
  - confusion.

Specific types of pain

Gastric pain, e.g. due to colic. Try a simple antacid or antiflatulent such as Gaviscon 10–20 ml p.r.n. Alternatively, use loperamide 2–4 mg q.d.s. orally or hyoscine hydrobromide tablets 300 µg t.d.s. sublingually.

Nerve pain, e.g. due to compression by a tumour mass or lymphadenopathy. Dexamethasone tablets 4–8 mg b.d. may reduce oedema around a tumour in the short term. Radiotherapy often provides relief for longer.

Muscle spasm This may be helped by the muscle relaxant baclofen 5–10 mg t.d.s. Alternatively, try diazepam 5–10 mg daily.

Bone pain, e.g. due to metastases. Opiate analgesics are the mainstay of treatment (see above). Radiotherapy and NSAIDs provide useful additional relief.

CONTROLLED DRUGS

For choices of drugs and dosages see pain, page 323.

Legal aspects
For prescribing opiates on the prescription form FP10 (GP10 in Scotland) a few simple rules have to be followed:

- Write the whole prescription in your own handwriting.
- The form, strength and dose of the drug must be stated, e.g. morphine sulphate elixir 10 mg/5 ml, 10 mg 4-hourly.
- The total amount of drug must be stated in words and figures, e.g. one hundred millilitres 100 ml.

For carrying controlled drugs in the black bag there are a few legal requirements:

- Keep a bound ledger to record the acquisition and administration of all controlled drugs. Use a different page for each form of drug. Record the amount, form and concentration of each drug and the dates acquired and used. Any difference between acquired and used drugs should equal what is left in the bag.
- If the black bag is left in the car it should be locked and the car should also be locked. Alternatively, controlled drugs can be kept in a separate locked container if left in a locked car.
- If stock goes out of date it can either be returned to the chemist or destroyed. Officially, the destroying of controlled drugs should be witnessed by a police officer, although this is rarely done in practice. There is controversy over the flushing of drugs down the toilet, a common procedure. The correct method is incineration (e.g. by using the sharps bin).

Ethical considerations
- In terminal care, the fear of addiction to opiates should not deter the doctor from adequately prescribing for pain relief.
- Addiction is unlikely to occur if the dose of opiate is adequate and given regularly.
- In the dying patient, pain and distress can prolong life by their stimulating effect on respiratory rate and arousal. Opiates relieve this distress and can allow patients to die peacefully, if somewhat earlier than they would

otherwise have done. This should not be considered a form of euthanasia. The dose of an opiate required to suppress the respiratory centre is much greater than that needed for pain relief.

VOMITING

Nausea and vomiting are common symptoms in terminal care.

Causes of vomiting in the terminally ill patient
- Drug side-effects, particularly chemotherapy drugs and opiates.
- Intestinal obstruction.
- Pain.
- Raised intracranial pressure, e.g. from cerebral metastases.
- Uraemia.
- Anxiety.
- Hypercalcaemia.

Diagnosis

History Ask about: • pain control • drug regimen • bowel/stoma function • headache • micturition.

Examination Look for:
- abdominal signs of obstruction
- papilloedema if raised intracranial pressure is suspected.

Investigations • U&E • calcium.

Management

 Treat the underlying cause if possible. Hospital/hospice admission is indicated if the cause of vomiting remains undiagnosed.

Reassure patients that their nausea can be treated.

Prescribing (e.g. for nausea associated with opiate analgesics):
- Prochlorperazine:
  – oral 5–10 mg t.d.s.
  – buccal 3–6 mg b.d.
  – suppository 5 and 25 mg

– injection 12.5 mg.
- Metoclopramide: tablets and injection 10 mg t.d.s.
- Domperidone:
  – tablets 10–20 mg 4–8-hourly
  – suppository 30–60 mg t.d.s.
- Cyclizine: injection 50 mg t.d.s. Cyclizine is useful when mixed with diamorphine in a syringe-driver as it can be given by subcutaneous infusion.

Side-effects
- Prochlorperazine and metoclopramide cause drowsiness and can cause acute dystonic reactions in younger patients.
- Domperidone is less sedating. Dystonia has been reported but is uncommon.
- Cyclizine can cause drowsiness, dry mouth and blurred vision.

Haematemesis This may be the final event in the course of a terminal illness.
   Diamorphine by i.m. injection can help relieve the acute distress to the patient.
   A red blanket on the bed helps to disguise the amount of blood being lost.

ANOREXIA

Anorexia is an inevitable feature of terminal care, as the appetite wanes and eating becomes too much of an effort.

> Anorexia is very common in the final few days of life and is often of more concern to the carers than to the patient. It may require no treatment, although attempting to improve the appetite may improve morale.

Management
- Exclude treatable causes:
  – drug side-effects
  – nausea
  – depression
  – abdominal obstruction
  – sore mouth, e.g. due to thrush.
- Simple measures:
  – give small helpings of food
  – use a small plate
  – suggest alcohol as an aperitif.

- Drug treatment:
  - prednisolone E/C tablets 5 mg t.d.s.
  - alternatively, dexamethasone 2–4 mg daily.

> It is rarely justifiable to use steroids simply to boost appetite, although steroids prescribed for other indications will improve overall well-being, including the appetite.

ANXIETY

Anxiety in the terminally ill may manifest itself as restlessness, confusion, agitation, depression or anger.

Diagnosis

History Ask about:
- symptoms common to terminal care, e.g. pain, vomiting, dyspnoea, constipation, anorexia
- psychosocial problems, e.g. distressed relatives, fear of dying or suffering, fear of hospitalisation
- free-floating anxiety; also pre-existing anxiety states
- drug side-effects.

Management
- Treat the underlying cause if possible.
- Give regular support and reassurance.
- Recognise anxiety and depression.
- Involve the district nurse, Marie Curie nurse, MacMillan nurse, and hospice or social worker, if appropriate, at an early stage.

Prescribing
- Antidepressants, e.g. imipramine 25 mg nocte, increased by 25 mg nocte at weekly intervals to a maximum dose of 150–200 mg.
  The side-effects of tricyclics include:
  - constipation
  - dry mouth
  - urinary retention
  - blurred vision
  - palpitations
  - drowsiness.

- Anxiolytics, e.g. chlorpromazine tablets or syrup 25 mg t.d.s increasing by 25 mg daily at weekly intervals until control is achieved.
  Side-effects include:
  – drowsiness
  – constipation
  – parkinsonism
  – postural hypotension.

Alternatively, use haloperidol 1–3 mg t.d.s., which is less sedating.
For short-term use in acute anxiety use diazepam 2 or 5 mg up to t.d.s.

 Cyclizine 50–150 mg or midazolam 40 mg can be given via a syringe-driver and can be mixed with diamorphine in the same syringe.

CONSTIPATION

Aim to prevent constipation in terminal care by prescribing laxatives in conjunction with opiate analgesics.

Causes of constipation in the terminally ill include: • opiate analgesics • decreased mobility • decreased fluid intake • anorexia • obstruction, e.g. due to tumour.

The overloaded colon may present with overflow diarrhoea. In this case liquefied stool bypasses a constipated segment of bowel. This possibility is worth bearing in mind when a patient on morphine presents with diarrhoea.

Management
(See also p. 118.)

- Always prescribe a laxative when giving opiate analgesics, e.g. the faecal softener and peristaltic stimulant co-danthramer 5–10 ml b.d.
- Exclude obstruction (absolute constipation, vomiting and distension, abdominal pain).
- If constipation occurs, an osmotic laxative such as lactulose 10 ml b.d. and a stimulant laxative such as bisacodyl 5–10 mg nocte can be given for 2 or 3 days.
- Stronger treatments may be necessary if the above measures fail, e.g. bisacodyl suppositories 10 mg (work within 20–30 minutes; this may cause griping abdominal pains). Alternatively, glycerol suppositories, docusate sodium or phosphate enemas may be useful.

COUGH

Cough is a common symptom in carcinoma of the bronchus.

 Some consequences of cough include insomnia and breathlessness. Carers may be disturbed at night.

Management
- Steam inhalations.
- Pholcodine linctus 10 ml 4-hourly.
- Morphine linctus 5 mg 4-hourly, increased until effective.

DEPRESSION

All terminally ill patients manifest depression at some stage of their illness. Depression in general is covered on page 294. Some features of depression are peculiar to the terminally ill.

Features of depression peculiar to terminal illness
- Ask about symptoms and look for signs of depression. The patient or carers may not volunteer these, leading to delayed diagnosis.
- Carer stress and depression are also common and should be sought.
- Features of depression may be masked by drugs used in terminal care, e.g. opiates and phenothiazines.
- Drug side-effects and interactions may complicate treatment, e.g. tricyclics and morphine both exacerbate constipation.
- District nurses, MacMillan nurses and Marie Curie nurses are an invaluable resource in the management of depression, both for identifying the condition and for supporting patients.

 The recently bereaved are at increased risk of suicide.

- The regular, close observation of the terminally ill patient by the GP should provide adequate opportunity for the detection and treatment of depression.

DYSPNOEA

Respiratory distress is common in terminal emphysema and carcinoma of the bronchus and may become a problem long before the patient is dying. Cheyne–Stokes breathing, on the other hand, is an almost universal feature of the last few hours of life, in anyone dying of malignant disease.

Management

Management of respiratory distress
- Exclude chest infection, pleural effusion and bronchospasm.
- Relieve the distress of dyspnoea with oral morphine 5 mg 4-hourly, increasing as necessary.
- Alternatively, use diazepam 5–10 mg daily.

Management of excessive respiratory secretions Excessive respiratory secretions are the cause of the 'death rattle' heard during the last few hours of the dying patient's life.

Give hyoscine or atropine injection (s.c. or i.m.) 600 μg t.d.s. Repeat if necessary after 6 hours.

DEATH

Most GPs will be involved in confirming or certifying a death approximately every 2 months, more frequently in the winter.

Talking to relatives
See bereavement, page 333.

Confirming death
When called to attend a patient who has died, the first task is usually to confirm death. Examine for: • carotid pulse • heart sounds • general appearance • fixed, dilated pupils.

> If the death occurs in the middle of the night, but was expected by the relatives or nursing-home staff, the examination to confirm death can often be left until the morning. Otherwise, visit as soon as possible.

Who to inform
At the time of confirming death it may only be necessary to inform those present – usually the relatives, especially if the death was expected.

Other people may need informing under the following circumstances:

- Relatives: if requested by those present at death.
- Undertaker: if requested by relatives.
- Coroner, if:
  - the death is sudden or unexplained
  - a doctor has not attended within the preceding 14 days
  - the death may be due to industrial disease, or related to the deceased's employment
  - the death was violent, unnatural or suspicious
  - the death may be due to an accident
  - the death may be due to self-neglect or neglect by others
  - the death may be due to an abortion
  - the death occurred during an operation or before recovery from the effects of an anaesthetic
  - the death may be a suicide
  - the death occurred during or shortly after detention in police or prison custody.
- Out-of-hours the coroner may not be available, in which case call the police.

Other people may need informing, but this can be done from the surgery during the next working day if necessary:

- a doctor from another practice if a Cremation Form Part B is required
- the patient's usual doctor
- Primary Healthcare Team members, if involved
- practice receptionist, to de-register the patient and cancel appointment reminders.

Administration

Forms

Death certificate The death certificate can be completed if the cause of death is known and the patient has been seen within the preceding 14 days by the doctor. If more than 14 days have elapsed, discuss the case with the coroner, who will probably 'pass' it if the cause of death is known. If in doubt, phone the coroner. Indicate on the back of the death certificate that the coroner has been informed.

The death certificate, if completed, can be collected from the surgery by the relatives, who use it to register the death at the Registrar's Office. If the death is made a coroner's case, the coroner issues the death certificate.

Cremation form The cremation certificate can be filled in only by doctors who have seen the dead body. Two doctors are required. The Part B doctor must have been fully registered for 5 years or more, must be from a different practice and must have discussed the death with the Part A doctor. The cremation form should be given to the undertaker.

Fees A fee is paid by the undertaker for completing a cremation certificate, either Part A or Part B. No fee can be claimed for completing a death certificate.

BEREAVEMENT

See also breaking bad news, page 322.

Anniversaries can rekindle various stages of bereavement.

Bereavement can be experienced following a loss other than a death, e.g. loss of marriage, job, pregnancy, limb.

The stages of bereavement
- Shock.
- Denial.
- Anger.
- Acceptance.

As a rule of thumb, the first two stages should last no longer than 1 or 2 days. Any significant lengthening of these stages should alert the GP to the possibility of an abnormal bereavement. Stages three and four can take longer, sometimes months, to complete.

Management
Most patients appreciate continued support at this time. Encouraging patients to talk about their loss helps the grieving process.

Inform the patient about support groups, e.g. Cruse (see p. 385).

Enlist the help of others. The district nurse, social worker, or a bereavement counsellor (e.g. from the hospice) may be useful.

⚠ There is an increased suicide risk in the recently bereaved. Involve the psychiatric team early in suspected abnormal grief or severe depression.

THE TREATMENT ROOM

EAR SYRINGING

Wax is formed from secretions from the ceruminous glands in the external ear canal. It has several functions, including lubrication, waterproofing of the ear and the prevention of infection. It becomes a problem when it is impacted and may lead to hearing loss.

Syringing should only be carried out by a nurse who has received appropriate training.

Olive oil ear drops (available OTC or on prescription), a few drops twice daily, should be used to soften wax for at least 7 days prior to syringing.

Very hard wax may need softening with sodium bicarbonate drops 5%. Commercial wax softeners are not recommended as they contain astringents which may irritate the skin of the ear canal and predispose them to otitis externa.

Reasons for syringing
- To improve the conduction of sound to the ear by the removal of impacted wax.
- To examine the external auditory meatus and tympanic membrane.

Before proceeding
- Take a careful history from the patient, regarding the presenting problem and previous medical ear history/allergies.
- Examine the ear with an auroscope with the patient seated. Look for signs of surgery behind the ear and signs of scaling or cracking of the skin.
- Examine the pinna, external meatus and scalp for abnormalities.
- Hold the auroscope like a pen, with the little finger resting against the patient's head to provide stability if the head is moved.
- Use the largest specula that will fit comfortably in the ear and gently insert the auroscope, pulling the pinna backwards and upwards in adults and backwards and downwards in children.
- Look for a cone of light, the long process of the incus and the short process of the malleus.
- Check the condition of the meatus as you remove the auroscope.

Contraindications for syringing
- No wax in the ear.
- Recent history of otalgia.
- Previous problems during syringing, e.g. faint.
- Discharging ear/chronic otitis externa.

Equipment for ear syringing
- Propulse pump.
- Waterproof cape and towel.
- Auroscope.
- A head mirror or light is recommended for a good view during the procedure.
- Water at 38°C.
- Trough or receiver.
- Jobson horne probe and cotton wool.
- Crocodile forceps.
- Tissues.

Procedure for ear syringing
- Check the previous history and any contraindication to the procedure.
- Explain the procedure to the patient and obtain informed consent.
- Ask the patient to sit in a chair with their head tilted towards the affected ear.
- Inspect the ear to be syringed with the auroscope.
- Put a protective cape, a towel and the receiver in position.
- Check that a light is in place, where applicable, and check the temperature of the water in the propulse reservoir (should be 38°C).
- Connect the tip to the holder until a 'click ' is felt.
- Set the pressure at the lowest setting.
- Run the water through for 10–20 seconds until warm (each time after you have stopped); this will also enable the patient to get used to the sound.
- Twist the jet tip in the right direction (5 minutes to the hour for the right ear and 5 minutes past the hour for the left ear).
- Warn the patient that you are about to start and remind them to keep still and that you will stop the procedure when asked.
- Straighten the meatus by pulling the pinna backwards and upwards, as described previously.
- Place the nozzle in the external entrance, switch on the machine and direct the stream of water along the roof of the meatus. Increase the pressure, to no more than the middle position, if the aural condition allows. A maximum of two reservoirs are used in any one procedure.
- Periodically inspect the meatus with the auroscope.
- After removal of wax or debris, dry mop using a Jobson horne probe and cotton wool (stagnation of water and abrasion of skin during the procedure predisposes to otitis externa).
- Record all findings and treatment.

- Past history of ear problems, e.g. perforated tympanic membrane.
- Grommets.
- Previous ear surgery.
- Likely uncooperative patient – age/dementia.
- The only 'hearing ear'.
- Unrepaired cleft palate.
- Medication, e.g. warfarin – take great care when using instruments.

 Syringing may cause discomfort, but should never cause pain. If the patient complains of pain, stop the procedure immediately.

Side-effects of syringing
- Otalgia.
- Vertigo.
- Tinnitus.
- Otitis externa.

The above should be short lived and the patient fully recovered in minutes.

Educate the patient on ear care
- Do not use cotton buds.
- Keep ears dry, washing the external area only.
- Wax is a normal product and not dirty.
- Wax is a problem only when it becomes impacted.
- Hearing aids may cause wax to impact and cause acoustic feedback (whistling).

Acknowledgement   This section on ear syringing was compiled with reference to the Aural Care Workshops, with the kind permission of Bernadette Mitchell.

VENEPUNCTURE

Venepuncture is carried out for two reasons:

- to obtain a blood sample for diagnostic purposes
- to monitor levels of blood components.

This is a routine procedure, but in order to carry it out safely the phlebotomist must have an understanding of: the relevant anatomy and physiology, the criteria for choosing the vein, the device to use, skin preparation and personal safety.

The sites of choice are the branches of the basilic vein, the cephalic vein and the median cubital vein in the antecubital fossa. These sizeable vessels are capable of providing copious and repeated blood specimens. The brachial artery and median nerve are very close by and must not be damaged.

The choice of vein must be that which is best for the individual patient. Injury or disease may prevent the use of a limb for venepuncture, i.e. the hemiplegic side of a patient following a stroke.

Factors influencing the dilation of veins include anxiety, temperature, mechanical irritation (good technique prevents trauma and reduces the likelihood of vein collapse) and the clinical state of the patient (e.g. dehydration or poor peripheral circulation as in heart failure).

The device commonly used to perform venepuncture for blood sampling is a closed vacuum container system, whereby the blood is transferred from the vein via a double-ended needle directly into the collecting tube. The flow will stop when the tube is filled to its vacuum capacity. The technique avoids the need for manual transfer from syringe to tube, thereby minimising the handling of blood.

Skin cleansing is generally considered to be of little value when performing venepuncture on a person with normally clean skin. Hygiene is important, however, as the skin is breached. The hands of the phlebotomist and the skin of the patient are potential sources of microbial contamination; therefore, good handwashing technique is essential.

With regard to personal safety, universal precautions are required when taking blood:

- every patient should be considered as a potential biohazard
- latex or vinyl gloves should be worn
- avoid needle-stick injury
- dispose of sharps and/or soiled equipment appropriately and safely (keep gloves on during this process and then dispose of gloves safely)
- protect cuts or other skin breaks on hands
- the phlebotomist must ensure they are immunised against hepatitis B.

Procedure for venepuncture

- Check the specimen request and select the appropriate tubes.
- Approach the patient in a confident manner and explain the procedure, consulting the patient on preferences and experiences related to previous venepuncture.
- Gather the necessary equipment.
- Position the patient in a suitable place, taking into account: lighting, ventilation, privacy, and nurse and patient safety and comfort. Where possible, request the patient to sit upright, although in those with a history of fainting it is best to position the patient lying on a couch.

Continued

Procedure for venepuncture – *continued*

- Examine both arms and choose the most suitable according to the aforementioned criteria.
- Fully extend the chosen arm and position it downwards. The arm should be supported, comfortable and relaxed.
- Wash your hands.
- Assemble the device.
- Apply a tourniquet above the elbow, ensuring that it does not obstruct the arterial flow.
- The veins may be tapped lightly.
- Select the vein.
- Put gloves on.
- Anchor the vein by applying manual traction to the skin just below the proposed insertion site.

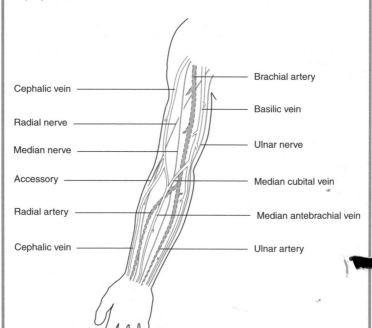

Cephalic vein

Radial nerve

Median nerve

Accessory

Radial artery

Cephalic vein

Brachial artery

Basilic vein

Ulnar nerve

Median cubital vein

Median antebrachial vein

Ulnar artery

Continued

Procedure for venepuncture – *continued*

- Hold the assembled device, with the needle bevel upwards, between thumb and index finger, penetrate the skin and insert the needle into the vein, smoothly at an angle of approximately 15°. Level off the needle after entry, so it is flush with the skin.
- Advance the needle approximately 1 cm into the vein if possible.
- Once satisfied that the needle is safely anchored, swap hands and, whilst supporting the device, press the tube home with the thumb of the free hand. Blood should then be drawn into the tube. Continue to hold the device until the tube fills; flow will stop automatically.
- Once the blood has begun to flow, release the tourniquet.
- Once the tube is filled, hold the device steadily with one hand, and with the other hand disengage the tube and gently agitate, but do not shake, to mix the blood and additive.
- Should more than one sample be required, remove the filled tube and replace with another immediately.
- Once all samples have been obtained, remove the needle.
- Place cotton wool over the puncture site and ask the patient to apply gentle pressure until the bleeding has stopped (approximately 1 minute; longer for those on warfarin or heparin).
- Inspect the puncture site and apply a clean swab, secured with tape.
- Dispose of sharps and soiled equipment safely.
- Check that the patient feels well and comfortable. They may need help with dressing or to lie down for a while.
- Label and pack tubes for transport to the laboratory.

WOUND MANAGEMENT

Key points in wound management
- An holistic assessment should be carried out initially. The wound should be reassessed regularly, as appropriate.
- Encourage good nutrition.
- Provide psychological support.
- Encourage adequate rest and sleep.
- Discourage smoking.
- Consider debridement of necrotic wounds.
- Consider systemic antibiotics if there is surrounding cellulitis.
- Prevent cross-infection.

Assessment

History

It is important when assessing a wound not to focus purely on the wound itself, but to consider the patient as a whole in order to avoid missing vital information that may influence wound healing.

The following factors should be considered:

- Lifestyle. Factors that may delay wound healing include:
  - poor nutritional state
  - smoking
  - increased alcohol intake
  - lack of sleep/rest
  - psychological factors (e.g. depression, stress, anxiety).
- Underlying disease.
- Age.

Classification of wounds

Wounds are generally classified by their colour, as follows:

- Black – indicates a necrotic wound, often with hard eschar present.
- Yellow – indicates slough.
- Green – indicates the presence of bacteria, but not always clinical infection. Bacteria can colonise a wound without delaying the healing process. The colour of discharge may vary according to the invading bacteria and may be yellow, green, red/brown or grey.
- Red – denotes granulation tissue, which is deep pink or red in colour. This is not always healthy tissue and may indicate wound infection or contamination with foreign bodies (e.g. fibres from dressings).
- Pink – pink epithelial tissue migrates from the wound edges and from undamaged hair follicles once the granulation tissue has reached the level of the surrounding skin.

Management

Wound cleansing

When cleansing a wound, several factors need to be considered:

- Cotton wool and gauze should be avoided and dressing materials should be sterile.
- Gloved hands are preferable to forceps, but be aware of the possibility of latex allergy.
- Cleansing reduces the bacterial count rather than removing bacteria.
- Complete elimination of bacteria is not a prerequisite to wound healing.
- Antiseptics can have toxic effects on microcirculation.
- Wiping the surface of a wound can damage granulation tissue.
- Surgical wounds should be cleaned with warm, sterile saline; all other wounds may be cleaned with warm tap water.

Choice of dressing

There is a lack of good-quality evidence for the effectiveness of wound dressings. However, it is widely accepted that a warm moist environment encourages healing and prevents tissue dehydration and cell death.

Dressings should:

- provide mechanical protection
- protect against secondary infection
- be non-adherent and be easily removed without trauma
- leave no foreign particles in the wound
- minimise excess exudate without allowing 'strike-through' to the surface of the dressing
- be cost-effective
- offer pain relief.

INFECTION CONTROL

Priorities are three-fold:
- detection of infection
- treatment of infection
- prevention of cross-infection.

Detection of infection

The following factors may indicate wound infection:

- new or increased levels of pain in or around the wound
- change in the appearance of the wound exudate
- granulation tissue that bleeds easily
- development of unpleasant odour
- localised inflammation around the wound
- non-healing
- increasing wound size
- cellulitis or oedema
- wound breakdown
- general malaise in the patient/fever

If there are signs of infection, consider taking a swab to identify the infecting organism.

Treatment of infection

This involves clinical decision-making related to the following:

- Systemic management – the use of oral antibiotics for wounds that are known to be clinically infected is preferable to attempting to manage the wound with a topical application.
- Use of antiseptics – a sound rationale is necessary for the cleansing of wounds with antiseptic solutions, as saline or clean water may be as effective.

Choice of dressing (always read the information contained in the dressing package)

Wound type	Treatment objective	Recommended primary products (in order of absorbency)	Recommended secondary products (in order of absorbency)
Necrotic	To remove/rehydrate black eschar	Hydrogel Hydrocolloid	Polyurethane foam dressing Hydrocolloid sheet Vapour-permaeble film dressing
Moist sloughy	To remove slough and provide a clean wound bed	As above Also consider alginate sheet or Cadexomer iodine dressing*	As above
Infected	To eradicate infection (antibiotics may be required) To remove excessive exudate and odour	Hydrocolloid fibrous dressing Alginate sheet dressing Cadexomer iodine dressing* Activated charcoal cloth with silver Povidone-iodine dressing Silver sulphadiazine cream	Absorbent pads Polyurethane foam dressing Absorbent perforated film dressing Low-adherent knitted viscose dressing
Granulating	To promote granulation and provide trauma-free healing	Hydrocolloid fibrous dressing Alginate sheet dressing Polyurethane foam Hydrocolloid sheet with absorbent granules Hydrocolloid sheet or gel Absorbent perforated film dressing Soft silicone wound contact dressing	Polyurethane foam Absorbent pads Hydrocolloid sheet

Cavity	To promote granulation and remove excessive exudate and odour To prevent premature wound closure	Hydrofibre dressing Alginate Polyurethane foam pads Activated charcoal cloth with silver Hydrogel Foam stent	Absorbent pads Polyurethane foam Hydrocolloid sheet
Epithelialising	To provide trauma-free healing To allow wound maturation	Polyurethane foam Low-adherent knitted viscose with silicone Hydrocolloid sheet Low-adherent knitted viscose dressing Soft silicone wound contact dressing Vapour-permeable film dressing	Absorbent pads
Fungating or malodorous	To remove excessive exudate and odour To avoid wound trauma	Activated charcoal cloth with silver Carbon dressing Cadexomer iodine dressing* Soft silicone wound contact dressing Topical metronidazole† Silver sulphadiazine cream	Absorbent pads Polyurethane dressing Hydrocolloid sheets

*Iodine dressings should be used with caution in patients with thyroid disease and those patients taking amiodarone.
†Topical metronidazole should be used with caution in patients on warfarin therapy.

- Topical management – the following preparations may be of some benefit:
  - silver sulphadiazine cream may reduce the bacterial load of the wound
  - cadexomer iodine is effective against a range of organisms, including *Staphylococcus aureus*
  - mupirocin is useful for the management of wounds colonised with MRSA (methicillin-resistant *S. aureus*)

Prevention of cross-infection

- MRSA is commonly spread by hand contact of the carers. Patients with MRSA in the community do not need to be isolated.
- Handwashing is most important to prevent the spread of infection.
- Gloves and an apron should be worn to perform a dressing.
- Paper covers should be used on the treatment room couch before use. After use the couch should be washed down with hot water and detergent, dried well and sprayed with 70% alcohol before the next patient.
- Patients with MRSA should preferably be treated at the end of a list.
- When carrying out any dressings it is essential to follow infection-control handwashing procedures before and after dealing with wounds.
- Dispose of used dressings in accordance with infection-control guidelines.

SURGICAL WOUND DRESSINGS

The purposes of wound dressings in this instance are to:

- absorb wound exudate
- protect the wound from injury
- protect the wound from bacterial infection.

 If the wound does not need dressing for any of these reasons, then a dressing may be safely omitted.

DONOR SITE DRESSINGS

Donor sites are superficial wounds, and left undisturbed should heal in 8–14 days.

Dressing is not recommended. Paraffin gauze may adhere to the wound bed, as it dries out too quickly, causing damage on removal. Film dressings are not recommended as they cannot deal with exudate.

Recommended dressings

- Calcium alginate dressings – have the most haemostatic properties.
- Polyurethane dressings – are hydrophilic, with low adherence to the wound surface and their waterproof outer layer prevents strikethrough.

- Soft silicone dressings – are non-adherent, but should be covered with a secondary dressing.

SUTURE AND CLIP REMOVAL

The timing of the removal of skin closures depends on the location on the body.

Guidelines
- Neck and head 3–5 days.
- Chest and abdomen 5–7 days.
- Lower extremities 7–10 days.
- Or on the instructions of the surgeon.

Note: Healing can be hindered by medical condition or obesity, infection or treatments such as steroids.

There is no rationale for removing alternate clips on consecutive days.

Dissolvable sutures are usually clear and it is usually only necessary to remove the knotted ends after 10 days.

If clips or staples are to be removed by a practice or district nurse, the appropriate tool should be given to the patient to take home.

SPECIFIC WOUNDS

For the treatment of burns, cuts and abrasions, skin tears in the elderly, and animal bites, see management of minor injuries, page 349.

CAVITY WOUNDS

Cavity wounds should be probed with extreme caution in order to detect the extent of the wound. Infection can be difficult to diagnose as these wounds become readily colonised.

Suitable dressings
- Alginates are the dressing of choice. They are available in sheets, ropes and ribbons. They should be loosely packed in the wound. Most are easily removed by irrigating with saline; otherwise they are removed using forceps or a gloved hand.
- Other dressings that may be considered are:
  - hydrocolloid fibrous dressings
  - foam stent dressings
  - polyurethane foam dressings
  - hydrogels (suitable for lightly exuding, shallow wounds)
  - hydrocolloid paste and flat hydrocolloid sheets
  - cadexomer iodine.

Overgranulation, hypergranulation or proud flesh

This occurs when the granulation tissue continues to be produced after the cavity is filled and produces a red, raised gelatinous mass that protrudes above the level of the skin. This impairs healing.

Before commencing treatment, it is essential to exclude a diagnosis of carcinoma. If suspected, the patient can be referred to a dermatologist and a biopsy taken.

Management options
- Take no action – overgranulation may resolve.
- If hydrocolloids have been used, change to a simple non-adhesive dressing.
- Apply light pressure to the wound bed by using supplementary padding on top of the primary dressing.
- Apply Lyofoam directly to the overgranulated tissue.
- Silver nitrate is used in the form of a stick applied directly to the overgranulating tissue. This will stain the wound bed black and should not be used for prolonged periods as it is caustic.
- Topical application of a topical steroid cream or ointment, under medical supervision.

WOUND DEBRIDEMENT

When there is suspicion that necrosis may be due to vascular disease, no attempt should be made to debride the area.

Benefits of wound debridement:

- Wound healing is optimised.
- Potential for infection is decreased.
- Necrotic tissue may have a foul odour.
- Necrotic or devitalised tissue may conceal underlying fluid collection or abscesses.
- Wound healing is impaired in the presence of necrotic tissue.
- Debridement of non-viable tissue is important in the management of contaminated wounds.

Types of debridement
- Autolytic debridement – this uses the body's own enzymes to digest devitalised tissue. This may be supported by the application of moisture-retentive dressings such as semipermeable film, hydrocolloids, polyurethane foam, alginates or continuously moist gauze.
- Surgical/sharp debridement – this requires specialist education or medical supervision and may require a general anaesthetic for large areas.

Acknowledgement   This section on wound management was compiled with reference to the Oxfordshire Wound Management Guidelines, with the kind permission of the Tissue Viability Service.

MANAGEMENT OF MINOR INJURIES

The use of the term 'minor injury' is misleading as the patient rarely views the injury as minor. The key skill required by the nurse when managing injured patients is the recognition of what can be managed locally and what needs referral to a more appropriate healthcare service.

It is important that the nurse recognises his or her limitations in decision-making related to patient care, always remembering the NMC Code of Professional Practice.

Rapid assessment

When a patient arrives in the treatment room, a rapid assessment of their condition is required, following a strict routine. Although his would seem to be aimed at major trauma and illness, the principles need to be applied to all injured patients.

The Primary Survey and Resuscitation Phase

A Airway with cervical spine control.
B Breathing and ventilation.
C Circulation and haemorrhage control.
D Disability(neurological examination).
E Exposure.

Airway

The most important question to ask is: 'Is the airway open and patent or is it closed and obstructed?'. The nurse should be aware of basic airway management skills as part of his or her mandatory training.

Breathing and ventilation

An assessment of the patient's breathing should include:

- respiratory rate
- respiratory effort/chest movement
- auscultation and percussion.

Early recognition of breathing problems is essential. Frequent monitoring should be carried out and, if the patient is found not to be breathing, resuscitation procedures should be initiated immediately, and medical help sought.

Circulation and haemorrhage control

A rapid assessment of the patient's haemodynamic status is essential, as haemorrhage resulting from injury can have catastrophic results if the bleeding is not recognised and treated promptly.

The important clinical indicators are:

- level of consciousness

- skin colour
- pulse – quality, rate and regularity.

External bleeding can be controlled by direct pressure using a sterile dressing and universal precautions. Do not apply tourniquets.

Disability

A rapid assessment of the patient's level of consciousness is required. The AVPU mnemonic is useful.

***

The AVPU
A Alert.
V Responds to vocal stimuli.
P Responds to painful stimuli.
U Unresponsive.

***

Pupil size and reaction should also be recorded. Any decrease or fluctuation in the level of consciousness may indicate a problem. Alcohol and drugs may affect this.

Exposure/environment control

The patient will need to be exposed in order for them to be fully examined. Depending on the severity of the injury, the patient's dignity needs to be maintained and the patient needs to be kept warm in order to prevent hypothermia.

Identifying the mechanism of injury is a vital component of the initial assessment and history-taking process, as vital information about injury patterns and likely injuries may be identified.

Clear information about the mechanism will inform decision-making. For example:

- How did you fall? Did you invert or evert your ankle? (As the patient to demonstrate this with the uninjured leg.)
- When you fell, how did you land? (Evidence shows that certain mechanisms of injury are associated with certain injury patterns.)

Have a high index of suspicion. Beware:

- the injury that the mechanism does not explain
- the patient who has little memory of the mechanism
- the patient who seems very accident prone and describes repeated falls, burns, etc.

Consider:

- non-accidental injury
- domestic violence

Examples of commonly seen injury patterns

Mechanism	Injury patterns	Consider
Crush injury	Circulatory compromise	Analgesia
	Open or closed fractures	Tet Tox booster/immunisation
	Skin and nail intact?	
	Extensive soft tissue damage?	
Inversion injury to ankle	Fractured tibia/fibula	History of weight-bearing at the time
	Associated fracture of the head of the fibula?	
	Open or closed?	
	Skin Integrity	
	Circulatory compromise	
	Soft tissue injury	Physiotherapy referral
Road traffic accident: patient in car	Cervical/lumbar spinal injury	Immobilise neck
	Fractured femur/ankle	High index of suspicion regarding impact velocity
	Head injury from glass?	Glass in wound/eyes?
Road traffic accident: pedestrian	Fractured tibial plateau	
	Head injury?	
	Internal injuries	

- deliberate self-harm
- elder abuse.

History

The history of an injury should always include:

- time of injury
- mechanism of injury
- cause of injury
- where it happened
- who was involved
- what happened next
- any significant past medical history, medications or allergies.

Notes should always include:

- date and time
- history
- physical findings

- investigation
- diagnosis
- treatment
- outcome or disposal
- signature (unless notes are computerised).

Examination

- Look – inspect the wound thoroughly in a good light. If there is a flap, note the colour of the skin, which may give an indication of flap viability. Assess the depth of the wound; consider drawing or photographing rather than describing a wound.
- Move – assess the anatomical function, the neurological function and the circulatory function around and distal to the wound.
- Feel – palpate gently around the wound to assess for the presence of a foreign body.

Management

Unless the patient is being transferred, follow the seven steps shown below.

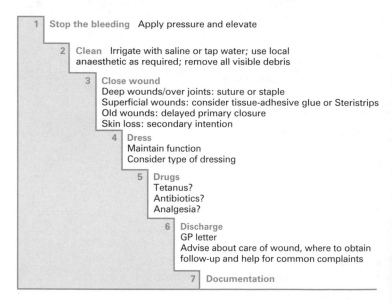

1   Stop the bleeding   Apply pressure and elevate

2   Clean   Irrigate with saline or tap water; use local anaesthetic as required; remove all visible debris

3   Close wound
Deep wounds/over joints: suture or staple
Superficial wounds: consider tissue-adhesive glue or Steristrips
Old wounds: delayed primary closure
Skin loss: secondary intention

4   Dress
Maintain function
Consider type of dressing

5   Drugs
Tetanus?
Antibiotics?
Analgesia?

6   Discharge
GP letter
Advise about care of wound, where to obtain follow-up and help for common complaints

7   Documentation

If the wound was caused by glass, an X-ray is indicated. If it is a dog bite there is a risk of infection.

Wounds sustained in a dirty environment such as a farm or garden will need more time spent on cleansing. Where there has been a delay of more than 6 hours (12 hours for the face) in seeking help, consider delayed primary closure and the potential for infection. Look for associated injuries. Warfarin may explain prolonged bleeding, and long-term steroid use will delay healing.

Refer to specialist medical staff if:

- there is evidence of damage to underlying structures
- there are signs of systemic infection
- the wound requires debridement
- there are deep wounds over joints
- the wound requires specialist closure (i.e. lip margins, around the eye)
- the wound contains foreign bodies that are not easily removed.

SPECIFIC WOUNDS

Pretibial lacerations
- Note the viability of the skin flap – is it pink with a good blood supply, or dusky?
- Avoid suturing, especially in the elderly.
- Where possible use self-adhesive strips and cover with a non-adherent dressing. Apply Tubigrip to the affected limb.

Consider referral to plastics if there:

- is a non-viable large flap
- is a large non-evacuable haematoma
- is damage to underlying structures
- is a history of poor healing
- are distal based flaps.

All pretibial lacerations should be followed up and the patient should be encouraged to elevate the affected limb.

Human and animal bites
Human bites are potentially more serious than animal bites, as the human mouth is heavily contaminated by bacteria and therefore these wounds have a high risk of infection.

All bites require:

- irrigation with normal saline or water
- application of a non-adhesive dressing
- assessment of tetanus status
- careful consideration regarding closure or not.

Consider:

- Potential infection with HIV/hepatitis B. Refer if the biter is high risk.
- Antibiotics may be indicated, but clinicians increasingly suggest observing for signs of infection and commencement of antibiotics if infection is confirmed.

Refer deep facial bites that may involve underlying structures to maxillofacial surgeons.

Discharge with wound advice, elevation, prescription if necessary, referral letter as required and a follow-up appointment.

Stings and insect bites

Assess for systemic and local reaction.

If the patient experiences anaphylaxis, summon medical help and consider emergency treatment according to local policy.

Treatment involves removal of the sting, if still present. Localised inflammation, cellulitis and swelling may need further medical treatment.

Nail injuries

These include subungual haematomas produced by crushing injury, nail avulsion, ingrowing toe nails and disruption of the nailbed.

Assess the extent of the injury plus involvement of underlying tissues, excluding fracture of the terminal phalanx.

Treatment

- Subungual haematoma – trephine.
- Nail avulsion – consider extent of injury and refer if necessary.
- Refer – if there is extensive underlying tissue damage; an ingrowing toenail may need referral to a podiatrist.

It is always better to refer patients to A&E if you are unsure of the extent of their injury.

Head injuries

See page 290.

Soft tissue injury to the lower limb

Soft tissue injuries are common in the lower limb. Ankle stability is dependent on a complex structure of ligaments that are prone to strain in inversion or eversion injuries. Assess for possibility of bony injury, requiring an X-ray

---

The Apley 'look, feel, move' model
Look   Skin; soft tissue; bone
Feel   Skin; soft tissue; bone
Move   Active; passive; stability

The discharge advice given to patents with soft tissue injury is perhaps the most important aspect of care.

RICE method of soft tissue treatment

R Rest to combat pain and reduce swelling initially.

I Application of an ice pack for 10–15 minutes at a time, three to four times a day. Do not apply direct to skin.

C The use of a compression bandage to prevent further swelling.

E Elevation of the limb when at rest and overnight to reduce swelling.

Burns

Management principles

- Stop the burning process by removing the burn agent. In chemical burns, the affected area needs copious irrigation.
- Avoid infection by asepsis; this will maximise the chances of healing.
- Dress burns to exclude infection.
- Consider excision and grafting for full-thickness burns and some partial thickness burns, so refer early.
- Tetanus immunisation should be checked and covered, as with all wounds.
- Routine antibiotics are not needed. If a patient presents with an old burn that is infected, then treat with antibiotics.
- Early referral is needed for large and full-thickness burns.

Referral

- Burns involving >10% of total body surfaces in an adult.
- Burns involving >5% of total body surfaces in a child.
- Full-thickness burns of >1% of total body surface area.
- Serious burns of face, neck, scalp, hands, eyes, genitalia or perineum.
- Burns involving the airway.
- Significant smoke inhalation.
- Chemical and electrical burns.
- Circumferential burns to the limbs, hands, feet, chest, abdomen, neck or face.
- Burns with existing medical problem.
- Any percentage injury in extremes of age.

Treatment of minor burns

First aid measures are to remove the source of the burn and to apply cold soaks. Immersion of the hand, foot, etc., into cold water is essential and may help with pain relief. Additional simple analgesia may be required as minor burns are often very painful.

After initial assessment, the burn needs to be dressed to prevent infection.

Wound care

- Erythema needs no dressing; cooling the skin and moisturiser will suffice.
- Blisters are best left intact to form a natural dressing. If the blister is large and restricts movement, it can be aspirated under aseptic technique, leaving the roof of the blister intact.
- If the patient needs to be transferred, then cling film may be used.
- Silver sulphadiazine cream is useful under a non-adherent dressing.
- Dressings that restrict movement can have long-term consequences and should be avoided.

Eyes

 Specialist advice should always be sought where there is any concern with eye injuries.

History
Ask the patient:

- What they were doing at the time of injury.
- Whether they were wearing eye protection.
- Flying objects – was a grinder or chisel used? Consider penetrating injury.
- Were they welding? Could they have arc eye?
- Is it related to injury? Consider glaucoma, conjunctivitis.
- If there is visual disturbance, when did it occur?
- Chemical splash – what was it? When did it go in? Call the poisons unit.
- Urgent irrigation may be required, pre-examination.
- Consider use of anaesthetic eye drops to aid examination and reduce discomfort.

Assessment

- Visual acuity with a Snellen chart – standing 6 m away.
- Visual fields.
- Vision – burning, flashing lights (detached retina?).

Examine the:

- bony orbits
- eyelids – invert upper eyelid and wipe with a damp cotton bud
- conjunctiva
- cornea
- iris
- pupil reaction (fixed, oval pupils may indicate glaucoma).

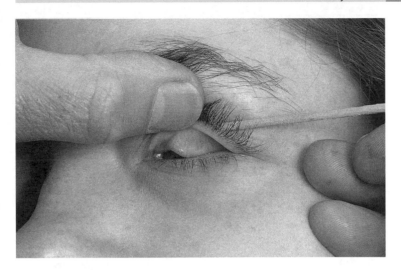

Everted upper lid (reproduced with permission from Maclean H 2002 The eye in primary care, Butterworth-Heinemann/Update.

Look for:

- Foreign bodies, blisters, inflammation, red eye, rashes around the eye, irregular pupils, blood around the eye, blood associated with hyphaema, hard eyeball, fixed pupils, photophobia.
- Note associated systemic illness or associated injuries.

Flourescein stain with a blue light will demonstrate corneal abrasions.

Referral
- Embedded foreign bodies.
- Corneal abrasion.
- Meibomiam cyst.
- Conjunctivitis lasting more than 1 week.
- Chemical splash – irrigate. Refer if appropriate.
- Patients who are haemodynamically unstable.
- Penetrating injury.
- Hyphaema.
- Blunt trauma to eye.
- Acute glaucoma.
- Suspected retinal tears.

If in doubt, call specialists for advice.

LEG ULCERS

Local leg ulcer strategy must be referred to, but the following provides a guide to management.

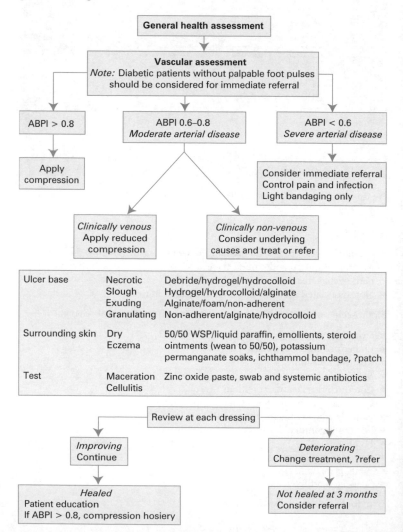

General health assessment

Vascular assessment
Note: Diabetic patients without palpable foot pulses should be considered for immediate referral

ABPI > 0.8

Apply compression

ABPI 0.6–0.8
Moderate arterial disease

ABPI < 0.6
Severe arterial disease

Consider immediate referral
Control pain and infection
Light bandaging only

Clinically venous
Apply reduced compression

Clinically non-venous
Consider underlying causes and treat or refer

Ulcer base	Necrotic	Debride/hydrogel/hydrocolloid
	Slough	Hydrogel/hydrocolloid/alginate
	Exuding	Alginate/foam/non-adherent
	Granulating	Non-adherent/alginate/hydrocolloid
Surrounding skin	Dry	50/50 WSP/liquid paraffin, emollients, steroid
	Eczema	ointments (wean to 50/50), potassium permanganate soaks, ichthammol bandage, ?patch
Test	Maceration	Zinc oxide paste, swab and systemic antibiotics
	Cellulitis	

Review at each dressing

Improving
Continue

Deteriorating
Change treatment, ?refer

Healed
Patient education
If ABPI > 0.8, compression hosiery

Not healed at 3 months
Consider referral

Types of leg ulcer

Type	Prevalence	Example of cause
Venous	70–90%	Deep vein thrombosis Varicose veins
Arterial	5–20%	Peripheral vascular disease Embolism
Neuropathic	5%	Diabetes mellitus Alcoholic neuropathy
Vasculitis	2–5%	Rheumatoid arthritis Polyarteritis
Trauma	≥2%	Laceration Inexpert bandaging
Haematological	1%	Sickle cell anaemia Thalassaemia Polycythaemia Leukaemia
Neoplastic	1%	Squamous cell carcinoma Basal cell carcinoma

Note: Ulcers may be associated with one or more of these causes. Up to 50% of patients with venous ulcers, over the age of 70 years also have arterial impairment.

Assessment
- The patient's general health should be assessed initially, and at 3-month intervals if not healing.
- The vascular state of the limb should be assessed.
- Ulcer size and wound state should be documented to monitor progress.
- A Doppler assessment must be carried out in each case and repeated 3-monthly, if compression is used.

Vascular (Doppler assessment)
A Doppler assessment should always be carried out prior to the application of compression therapy.

Doppler ultrasound detects the flow of blood in the blood vessels. It consists of a transducer (probe) that is attached to an audio unit. The probe should be used in conjunction with a coupling gel, which aids the transmission of ultrasound. The recommended probes are:

- 8 MHz for normal sized limbs
- 5 MHz for obese/oedematous limbs.

Arteries   Healthy arteries have a strong pulsating sound consisting of three phases (triphasic), but sometimes only two phases (biphasic) can be heard. It is important that practitioners recognise the normal pulsatile sound.

Veins   Veins do not pulsate and give a continuous 'whooshing' or 'roaring' sound.

Procedure
It is recommended that only staff who regularly use Doppler ultrasound and have received training and regular updating should carry out this procedure.

- The patient should be resting for 15–20 minutes, lying flat or as flat as possible, with their legs as horizontal as possible, and relaxed. A patient history may be taken during this time.
- Record the position of the patient.
- Place the sphygmomanometer cuff around the top of the arm. Palpate the pulse and apply ultrasound gel.
- Hold the Doppler probe between the forefinger and thumb at an angle of 45° and place it over the brachial pulse.
- Inflate the cuff until the Doppler sound disappears; slowly deflate the cuff until the sound returns. This is the brachial systolic pressure. Check the reading in each arm twice, leaving a time delay between each reading. Record the highest pressure reading.
- Palpate one of the arteries of the foot – usually the dorsalis pedis, but the posterior tibial, the peroneal or the anterior tibial may be used.
- Place the sphygmomanometer cuff around the ankle above the malleoli. If an ulcer is present, cover it with a low-adherent dressing with a sheet of polythene over the top.
- Inflate the cuff, keeping the probe where a strong pulse can be heard. Once the pulse signal disappears, gradually deflate the cuff until the sound returns. This is the ankle systolic pressure.
- Repeat the procedure using a different foot artery, usually the posterior tibial. Record the highest reading.

Calculating the ABPI
Spuriously high Doppler readings are sometimes obtained in patients with diabetes and in patients with calcified arteries. Doppler readings should therefore be used to confirm observations.

Method   Divide the ankle pressure reading by the brachial pressure reading:

$$\text{ABPI} = \frac{\text{Highest ankle systolic pressure}}{\text{Highest brachial systolic pressure}}$$

For example, with an ankle systolic pressure of 100 mmHg and a brachial systolic pressure of 140: ABPI = 100/140 = 0.71.

Interpretation of the ABPI
- Patients with an ABPI ≥ 0.8 may have compression bandaging or hosiery.
- Patients with an ABPI of 0.6–0.8 have moderate arterial disease. The assessment should indicate whether the ulcer is clinically venous, in which case reduced compression may be used; or clinically non-venous, in which case the underlying causes need to be considered. Referral is an option, especially for patients with diabetes.

> **Patients with an ABPI < 0.6 have severe arterial disease. Immediate referral should be considered. Retention bandages only should be applied.**

Management

> Compression is the most important factor in healing venous ulcers. No particular method of high compression has been shown to be superior. Where there is significant arterial disease, no compression should be applied.

- Padding under compression improves comfort and protects bony prominences.
- Warmed tap water is adequate for cleansing.
- The appropriate dressing will provide the optimum environment for wound healing; however, no dressings on their own have been shown to enhance the healing rate of venous ulcers. Dressings should be chosen to take into account comfort, frequency of attendance and cost-effectiveness.
- If infected, take a swab. If appropriate, prescribe oral antibiotics, e.g. flucloxacillin, or, if foul smelling, metronidazole. Treat cellulitis with oral penicillin or erythromycin.
- Care should be taken of the surrounding skin.

Choice of dressings
It is the application of compression, not the dressing type, that will encourage a leg ulcer to heal and help to reduce exudate.

Dressing choices for different conditions of ulcers are given on page 362.

Monitoring
- Ulcer healing and management should be considered at each dressing.
- Patients in compression should have their ankle brachial pressure index (ABPI) checked at 3-month intervals.
- Patients with ulcers not showing signs of improvement within 3 months should be considered for referral.

Condition of ulcer	Objective	Treatment choice
Necrotic Localised death of tissue	To rehydrate/consider removal of black eschar	Surgical debridement, hydrogel/hydrocolloid
Sloughy Soft yellow necrotic tissue that separates from healthy tissue	To remove slough and provide a clean wound for granulation	Hydrogel/hydrocolloid, Cadexomer iodine paste, alginate, maggot therapy
Exuding Discharge of serum and cells, mostly leucocytes from the open wound	Manage levels of exudate by appropriate absorbtion	Non-adherent dressing, hydrocolloids, foam dressings, alginates
Granulating The outgrowth of new capillaries and connective tissue cells from the surface of an open wound	Promote granulation and provide trauma-free healing	Non-adherent dressings, hydrocolloids, alginates and foam dressings
Epithelialising Development of epithelium (the final stage in wound healing)	Provide trauma-free healing to allow wound maturation	Non-adherent dressings, hydrocolloids, polyurethane foam

Aftercare of healed venous leg ulcers

- Educate patients to care for their skin. The use of simple emollients such a 50/50 ointment helps to prevent dryness.
- Advise patients not to expose the limb to extremes of hot or cold.
- Advise on active exercise in mobile patients and passive exercise for the less mobile, i.e. foot flexions/extensions and rotation to prevent fixed ankle joints and aid venous return. Discourage standing for prolonged periods.
- Encourage patients to put their legs up as high as possible every time they sit down. This aids venous return and prevents oedema.
- Treatment of varicose veins may reduce recurrence in cases where the local oedema leads to thinning of the overlying skin.
- Stress the importance of well-fitting shoes, especially in patients who are at risk of foot ulceration due to ischaemia or neuropathy (e.g. diabetes).
- Advise on keeping weight down.
- Physiotherapy may be beneficial, e.g. exercises, gentle massage and local ultrasound.
- Consider the use of diuretics and analgesics.

Compression hosiery follow-up
See patients every 3 months for repeat Doppler readings and follow-up.

Recurrence
If recurrence occurs, the assessment process should be repeated. Each new episode of care should be managed independently from the last.

REFERENCES

Wound management

Hampton S (1997) Wound assessment. *Professional Nurse,* Study Supplement **12**: 12.

Miller M (1996) Wound cleansing in the community. *Nurse Prescriber*, June: 25–28

Thomlinson D (1987) To clean or not to clean? *Nursing Times*, **83**(9):71–75

Young T (1996) Methicillin resistant *Staphylococcus aureus. Journal of Wound Care*, **5**(10):475–477.

Management of minor injuries

Apley AG, Solomon L (1995) Apley's system of orthopaedics and fractures, 7th edn. Butterworth Heinemann, Oxford.

Bird D (1999) Transferring the thermally injured. *Emergency Nurse*, **7**(6):14–17.

Resuscitation Council (UK) (1998) Advance life support manual. Resuscitation Council UK, London.

Wardrope J, English B (1998) Musculo-skeletal problems in accident and emergency medicine. Oxford university Press, Oxford.

Management of leg ulcers

Cornwall J et al. (1989) The assessment, management and prevention of leg ulcers. *Care of the Elderly*, **2**.

Douglas WS, Simpson NB (1995) Guidelines on the management of chronic leg ulceration. *British Journal of Dermatology*, **113**:446–452.

DRUG MONITORING

Several drugs used in general practice require long-term monitoring in addition to the routine clinical follow-up of patients.

WARFARIN

Measurement INR (international normalised ratio) – the ratio of the patient's prothrombin time to the laboratory standard. Appropriate INR ranges:

- 2.0–2.5 for:
  - prophylaxis of deep-vein thrombosis.
- 2.5 for:
  - deep-vein thrombosis
  - pulmonary embolus
  - mitral stenosis with embolism
  - atrial fibrillation
  - tissue prosthetic heart valves.
- 3.0–4.5 for:
  - recurrent deep-vein thrombosis
  - recurrent pulmonary embolus
  - mechanical prosthetic heart valves.

Values are often recommended in hospital discharge letters, or see *British National Formulary*.

Duration of treatment Life, for all conditions except pig heart valve replacements and single episodes of deep-vein thrombosis or pulmonary embolus (3 months). Anticoagulation can also often be discontinued if haemorrhage occurs, e.g. from a bleeding peptic ulcer.

Starting dose 10 mg daily for 2 days, then between 3 and 9 mg daily according to the INR.

Frequency of measurement
- Prior to starting treatment.
- Daily initially, until the desired range is achieved (usually 3 days), then every 2 or 3 days. Thus, if commencing warfarin treatment in general practice, start on a Monday. Intervals increase as a stable dose is achieved. Aim for INR testing every 4–6 weeks once stable. Test more frequently if the INR is too high or too low, or following a change of dose.

LITHIUM

Measurement Serum drug level.
- Take blood 12 hours after the last dose.

Therapeutic range
- 0.8–1.2 mmol/l in acute mania.
- 0.4–1.0 mmol/l in manic depression.

Frequency of measurement
- 1 week after any change of dose.
- 3-monthly as a routine.
- More frequently if toxicity is suspected by:
  – nausea, vomiting, diarrhoea
  – muscle weakness, confusion
  – ataxia, dysarthria
  – arrhythmias, renal impairment.

Also measure C&E and TFTs annually to exclude hypothyroidism and renal impairment.

THEOPHYLLINE

Measurement Serum drug level.
- Measure 8 hours after the last dose (12 hours for modified release formulations).

Therapeutic range
- 55–110 µmol/l

Frequency of measurement
- 2–3 days after a change of dose.
- Routine measurements are unnecessary.
- Check levels if:
  – toxicity is suspected due to: nausea and diarrhoea, insomnia, tachycardia and arrhythmia
  – asthma control deteriorates
  – the patient gives up smoking
  – i.v. aminophylline is contemplated.

DIGOXIN

Measurement Serum drug level.
- Take blood 12 hours after the last dose.

Therapeutic range
- 1.0–2.6 nmol/l.

Frequency of measurement
- 8 days after any change of dose.
- Routine serum drug levels are unnecessary.
- Aim to control the ventricular rate <100/minute without side-effects.

- Measure drug level if toxicity is suspected due to:
  – anorexia, nausea, vomiting
  – confusion
  – arrhythmia.

  Also measure U&E if toxicity is suspected, as hypokalaemia potentiates the effect of digoxin.

THYROXINE

Measurement TSH (thyroid stimulating hormone).
- The timing of the sample is not important.

Therapeutic range
- 0.5–5.0 mU/l.

Frequency of measurement
- 1 month after a change of dose.
- Routine testing is not necessary, although some authorities advise annual testing.
- Measure the TSH and T4 and T3 if under- or overtreatment is suspected.
- Aim to maintain a euthyroid status.
- Reduce the dose of thyroxine if the TSH is below 0.08 mU/l.

PHENYTOIN

Measurement Serum drug level.
- The timing of the sample is not important.

Therapeutic range
- 40–80 µmol/l.

Frequency of measurement
- 7–10 days after each change of dose.
- Routine drug level measurement is unnecessary.
- Aim to control fits without side-effects. Therefore, measure levels if:
  – toxicity is suspected due to: nystagmus, ataxia or dysarthria
  – fits occur.
- If the serum drug level is <20 µmol/l, increase the daily dose by 100 mg.
- If the serum drug level is 20–60 µmol/l, increase the daily dose by 50 mg.
- Also measure FBC as appropriate (risk of agranulocytosis).

METHOTREXATE (and other immunosuppressants)

Measurement FBC, C&E and LFT.

Frequency of measurement Prior to treatment. Then weekly until therapy stabilised, then 3-monthly (there is a risk of agranulocytosis).

ACE INHIBITORS

Measurement C&E.

Frequency of measurement Prior to treatment, at 2 weeks and at every increase of dose (there is a risk of hyperkalaemia), then annually.

STATINS

Measurement LFT.

Frequency of measurement Prior to treatment, within 1–3 months of starting treatment, and thereafter at intervals of 6 months for 1 year.

DIURETICS

C&E 6-monthly (hypo- or hyperkalaemia).

SULPHASALAZINE

FBC and LFT monthly for the first 3 months (marrow suppression and liver toxicity).

GOLD

FBC and urinalysis for blood and protein prior to every injection (marrow aplasia and immune complex nephritis).

NURSE PRESCRIBING

The development of nurse prescribing within the UK has progressed slowly, but the implementation of the NHS Plan (DoH 2000) has begun to foster a culture of accesss to services and role devlopment to meet health needs. One such development is the extension of prescribing powers for nurses and other health professionals. In conjuction with this, amendments have been made to the law so that this may be carried out in a framework of professional accountability.

The Crown Report (DoH 1999) recommended that prescribing rights be extended to all groups of currently registered nurses. It identified two potential types of prescribing:

- Independent – which would assume full care and treatment of the patient from presentation.

- Dependent – now known as 'supplementary', which would assume full responsibility for the care of and prescribing to patients whose condition had been diagnosed by a medical practitioner.

Following a DoH consultation, in 2001 it was announced that suitably qualified nurses should be able to prescribe for a range of conditions in four therapeutic areas:

- minor illness
- minor injuries
- health promotion
- palliative care.

The medicinal products are designated in the *Nurse Prescriber's Extended Formulary* (NPEF) and comprise 140 prescription-only medicines (POMs), licensed for specific conditions within the four therapeutic areas. An outline curriculum was prepared by the former English National Board (ENB), with specific learning outcomes (DoH 2002).

The course is delivered over 3–6 months, with 25 days of classroom contact at an institute of higher education. In addition, students are required to spend 12 days in a practice setting to undertake supervised prescribing practice mentored by an appropriately qualified medical practitioner. Further amendments were made to the Health and Social Care Act in April 2003 to enable nurses and pharmacists to practice supplementary prescribing. Most universities have now amended their curriculum to incorporate supplementary prescribing.

Supplementary prescribing is a tripartite agreement between a patient, a supplementary prescriber and a medical practitioner to implement an agreed individual clinical management plan (CMP). The medical practitioner who is accountable for the patient diagnosis, and the supplementary prescriber, draw up the CMP. The CMP is a legal requirement for supplemantary prescribing to take place; it is patient specific and defines the parameters of treatment.

The supplementary prescriber is then responsible for the review of that diagnosis and may then prescribe appropriate medicinal products, which are outlined in the CMP for a specified period of time. There are no legal restrictions on the conditions that can be managed and no specific formulary other than all medicines prescribable by a medical practitioner on the NHS. It is considered that supplementary prescribing may be most approriate for chronic conditions.

References

DoH 1999 Review of prescribing, supply and administration of medicines. Crown 2. The Stationery Office, London.

DoH 2000 The NHS plan. The Stationery Office, London.

DoH 2002 Extending independent nurse prescribing within the NHS in England. The Stationery Office, London.

DoH 2003 Supplementary prescribing by nurses and pharmacists within the NHS in England – A guide for implementation. The Stationery Office, London.

PRIVATE MEDICAL EXAMINATIONS

Private medical examinations are often requested by either the patient or a third party. Examples include insurance company examinations, vocational driving licence examinations, sports examinations and examination of children in care.

Before agreeing to do the examination decide the following:

- How long will it take?
- Who is requesting it?
- Who is going to pay for it and what is the fee?
- Will I need extra equipment such as ECG, colour vision charts?

Set aside enough time. The receptionist can ask the patient to produce a specimen of urine before the appointment, if necessary, to save time.

Read through the questionnaire first to establish exactly what needs examining. Leave no blank spaces.

It is acceptable to tell the patient relevant findings of the examination, especially if these have implications for health. However, refrain from committing yourself on their likely insurance/licence risk – that is for the company to decide.

HIV testing forms part of some insurance examinations and is paid for separately by the companies. Make sure the patient is prepared to receive the result from the company and that they have contemplated the consequences of a positive result.

Keep a record of all earnings from private examinations and include the date done, patient name, company name, date the payment was received and the fee. This is for chasing up late payments and also for tax purposes.

PATIENT REPORTS

When asked to write a report on a patient, e.g. for a solicitor or an insurance company, several things make the job easier.

- Has the patient given written consent for details of their medical history to be revealed to the third party? If not, return the request asking for written consent.

- Often a pro forma questionnaire will accompany the request. This specifies the information needed and will usually be brief.
- Look at the patient's notes and computer record. Is there a copy of a recently completed questionnaire in the notes? If so, copy it, changing only those parts of the medical history that have occurred since the date of the last report.
- Summarised notes and computer summaries make preparing reports easier. Hospital letters may be helpful.
- If the patient has asked to see the report before it is sent, keep it for 21 days before posting it.
- Personal medical attendant's reports for insurance companies attract a fee agreed with the BMA and this is usually paid on receipt of the report by the company. Solicitors' reports do not specify a fee, and an invoice should be sent with the report, asking for payment by return of post. The fee should be based on the time taken to prepare the report and the BMA hourly rate for GPs.
- For all types of private reports keep a record of the date sent, patient name, company, the date payment was received and the fee. This will give an indication of who to send a reminder to for non-payment and also a running total for tax purposes.
- In many practices, the majority of the above tasks are undertaken by secretarial staff.

NOTIFIABLE DISEASES

The following diseases are statutorily notifiable by the GP if suspected or proven:

- anthrax
- cholera
- diphtheria
- dysentery (amoebic or bacillary)
- encephalitis (acute)
- food poisoning (microbiological or chemical)
- leprosy
- leptospirosis
- malaria
- measles
- meningitis
- meningococcal septicaemia (without meningitis)
- mumps
- ophthalmia neonatorum
- paratyphoid fever

- plague
- poliomyelitis (acute)
- rabies
- relapsing fever
- rubella
- scarlet fever
- smallpox
- tetanus
- tuberculosis
- typhoid fever
- typhus
- viral haemorrhagic fever
- viral hepatitis
- whooping cough
- yellow fever.

The most common is food poisoning.

UK HIV reporting is voluntary and confidential to the Communicable Disease Surveillance Control (see p. 385).

Notification is made to the Local Authority Environmental Health Department. Complete the form provided by the Environmental Health Office.

Notification by telephone is essential in suspected cases of food poisoning as it allows the Environmental Health Officer to take samples of faeces, vomit and food before the infection has gone.

A small fee is payable for each notification.

MANAGEMENT OF ANAPHYLAXIS

- Lie the patient in the left lateral position. If unconscious, insert an airway.
- Give adrenaline 1/1000 i.m. unless the carotid pulse is strong and the patient's condition is good (see below).
- Give oxygen, if available, by face mask.
- Start cardiopulmonary resuscitation, if appropriate.
- The following drugs may also be given:
  - chlorpheniramine maleate 5 mg i.v.
  - hydrocortisone 100 mg i.v. (to prevent further deterioration in severe cases).
- If there is no improvement in the patient's condition after 10 minutes, repeat the dose of adrenaline up to a maximum of three doses.
- Admit to hospital for observation.
- Report to the Committee on Safety of Medicines, if appropriate.

Adrenaline dosage
(Adrenaline 1/1000 = 1 mg/ml)

Adults	0.5–1.0 ml
<1 year	0.05 ml
1 year	0.1 ml
2 years	0.2 ml
3 years	0.3 ml
4 years	0.4 ml
5–10 years	0.5 ml

NORMAL HAEMATOLOGY VALUES

Acid phosphatase (total)		1–5 IU/l
Acid phosphatase (prostate)		0–1 IU/l
Alanine aminotransferase (ALT)		3–35 IU/l
Albumin		35–50 g/l
Alkaline phosphatase (adult)		30–300 IU/l
Aspartate aminotransferase (AST)		3–35 IU/l
Bilirubin		3–17 µmol/l
Calcium (total)		2.12–2.65 mmol/l
Cholesterol		3.9–6.0 mmol/l
Creatine kinase	Men	25–195 IU/l
	Women	25–170 IU/l
Creatinine		70–150 µmol/l
Folate (serum)		3–15 µg/l
Folate (red cell)		160–640 µg/l
Follicle stimulating hormone (FSH)		2–8 U/l
Gamma glutamyl transferase (γ-GT)	Men	11–51 IU/l
	Women	7–33 IU/l
Glucose (fasting)		3.5–5.5 mmol/l
Haemoglobin	Men	13.5–18 g/dl
	Women	11.5–16 g/dl

Iron	Men	15–31 µmol/l
	Women	14–30 µmol/l
Lactate dehydrogenase (LDH)		70–250 IU/l
Luteinising hormone (LH) premenopausal		6–13 U/l
Mean cell volume (MCV)		76–96 fl
Mean cell haemoglobin (MCH)		27–32 pg
Mean cell haemoglobin concentration (MCHC)		30–36 g/dl
Phosphate		0.8–1.45 mmol/l
Platelets		$150–400 \times 10^9$/l
Potassium		3.5–5.0 mmol/l
Prolactin	Men	< 450 U/l
	Women	<600 U/l
Prostate specific antigen (PSA)		0–4 ng/l
Protein (total)		60–80 g/l
Red cell count	Men	$4.5–6.5 \times 10^{12}$/l
	Women	$3.9–5.6 \times 10^{12}$/l
Sodium		135–145 mmol/l
Thyroid stimulating hormone (TSH)		0.05–6.0 mU/l
Thyroxine (T4)		70–140 nmol/l
Thyroxine (free)		9–22 pmol/l
Tri-iodothyronine (T3)		1.2–3.0 nmol/l
Total iron binding capacity (TIBC)	Men	45–70 µmol/l
	Women	44–74 µmol/l
Triglyceride		0.55–1.9 mmol/l
Urea		2.5–6.7 mmol/l
Uric acid	Men	210–480 µmol/l
	Women	150–390 µmol/l
Vitamin B_{12}		200–900 ng/ml
White cell count		$4–11 \times 10^9$/l

STANDARD GROWTH CHARTS

Data reproduced with permission of Castlemead Publications.

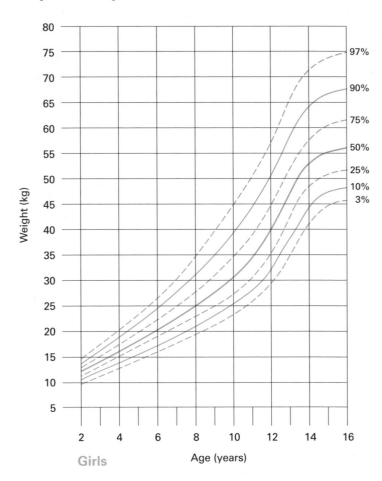

Girls

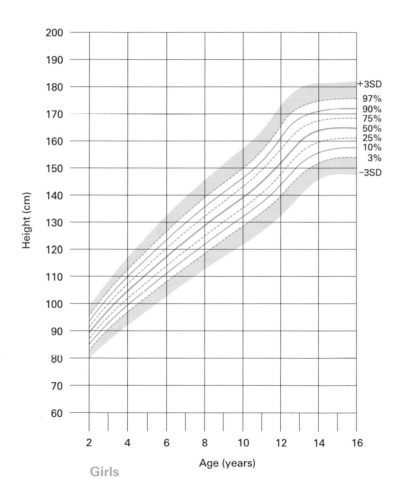

Girls

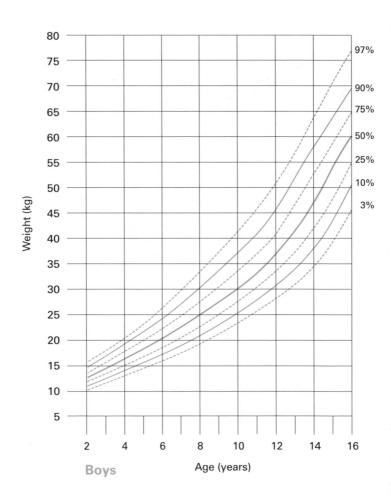

Boys — Age (years) vs Weight (kg)

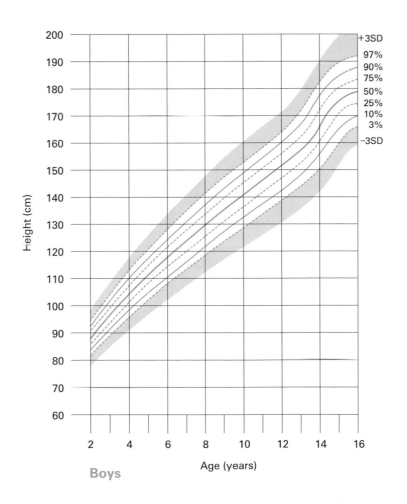

Boys

DERMATOMES

Reproduced with permission from Hayes PC, Mackay TW, Forrest EH 1996
Churchill's pocketbook of medicine, 2nd edn. Churchill Livingstone,
Edinburgh

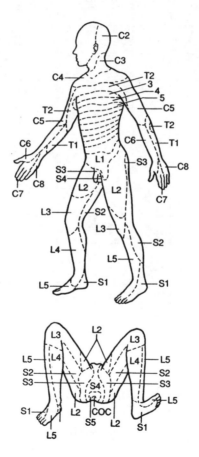

ADULT HEIGHT VERSUS WEIGHT CHART

From Garrow JS 1981 Treat obesity seriously. Churchill Livingstone, Edinburgh. Acknowledgements: Health Education Council, E Fullard, Oxford

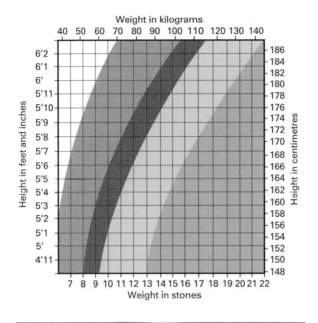

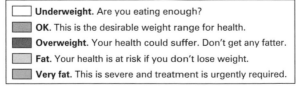

Underweight. Are you eating enough?

OK. This is the desirable weight range for health.

Overweight. Your health could suffer. Don't get any fatter.

Fat. Your health is at risk if you don't lose weight.

Very fat. This is severe and treatment is urgently required.

PEAK FLOW VALUE CHARTS

Reproduced with permission from Gregg I, Nunn AJ 1996 *British Medical Journal* 1973; 3:282

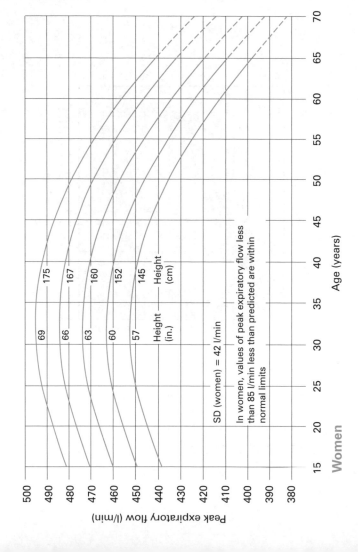

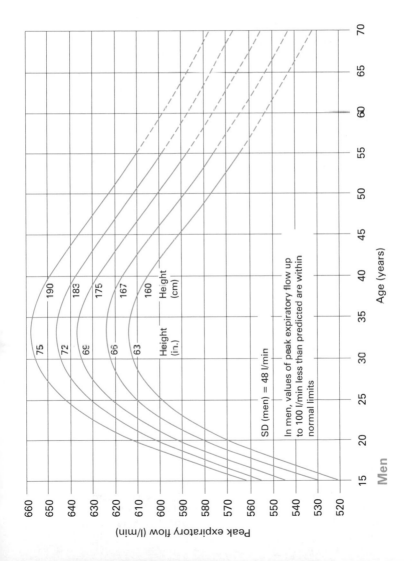

Men

Peak expiratory flow (l/min)

660
650
640
630
620
610
600
590
580
570
560
550
540
530
520

Age (years)

15 20 25 30 35 40 45 50 55 60 65 70

75
72
69
66
63
Height (in.)

190
183
175
167
160
Height (cm)

SD (men) = 48 l/min

In men, values of peak expiratory flow up to 100 l/min less than predicted are within normal limits

USEFUL ADDRESSES AND TELEPHONE NUMBERS

Age Concern
Astral House
1268 London Road
London SW16 4ER
Tel. 020 8765 7200 (Administration)
Tel. 0800 009966 (Helpline)

Alcoholics Anonymous (AA)
PO Box 1
Stonebow House
Stonebow
York YO1 7NJ
Tel. 01904 644026 (Administration)
Tel. 020 7833 0022 (London helpline)
(See telephone directory for local helplines)

Al-Anon Family Groups UK & Eire/Alateen
61 Great Dover Street
London SE1 4YF
Tel. 020 7403 0888

Alzheimer's Society
Gordon House
10 Greencoat Place
London SW1P 1PH
Tel. 020 7306 0606

Breast Cancer Care
Kiln House
210 New Kings Road
London SW6 4NZ
Tel. 020 7384 2984 (Administration)
Tel. 0808 800 6000 (Helpline)

British Acupuncture Association and Register
22 Hockley Road
Rayleigh
Essex M33 4RA
Tel. 01268 742534

British Association of Psychotherapists
37 Mapesbury Road
London NW2 4HJ
Tel. 020 8452 9823

British Association for Counselling and Psychotherapy
BACP House
35–37 Albert Street
Rugby
Warwickshire CV21 2SG
Tel. 0870 443 5252

British Heart Foundation
14 Fitzhardinge Street
London W1H 6DH
Tel. 020 7935 0185

British Homeopathic Association
Hahnemann House
29 Park Street West
Luton LU1 3BE
Tel. 0870 4443950

British Tinnitus Association
Ground Floor, Unit 5
Acorn Business Park
Woodseats Close
Sheffield S8 0TB
Tel. 0845 450 0321/0800 018 0527

CancerBACUP
3 Bath Place
Rivington Street
London EC2A 3JR
Tel. 0808 800 1234

Carers National Association
20–25 Glasshouse Yard
London EC1A 4JT
Tel. 020 7490 8818 (Administration)
Tel. 0345 573 369 (Helpline)

Cervical Stitch Network
'Fairfield'
Wolverton Road
Norton Lindsey
Warwickshire CV35 8LA
Tel. 01926 843223

Child Death Helpline
Great Ormond Street Hospital
Great Ormond Street
London WC1N 3JH
Tel. 020 7813 8551 (Administration)
Tel. 0800 282986 (Helpline)

Childwatch
19 Spring Bank
Hull
East Yorkshire HU3 1AF
Tel. 01482 325552

Communicable Disease Surveillance
Control
61 Collindale Avenue
London NW9 5EF
Tel. 020 8200 6868

CONI (Care of Next Infant)
Room C1
Stephenson Wing
Division of Child Health
The Children's Hospital
Western Bank
Sheffield S10 2TH
Tel. 0114 276 6452

Cruse Bereavement Care
Cruse House
126 Sheen Road
Richmond
Surrey TW9 1UR
Tel. 020 8939 9530 (Administration)
Tel. 0870 167 1677 (Helpline)

Cry-sis
BM Cry-sis
London WC1N 3XX
Tel. 020 7404 5011

Diabetes UK
10 Parkway
London NW1 7AA
Tel. 020 7424 1000

Dyslexia Institute
Park House
Wick Road
Egham
Surrey TW20 0HH
Tel. 01784 222300

Eating Disorders Association
103 Prince of Wales Road
Norwich NR1 1DW
Tel. 0870 770 3256 (Administration)
Tel. 0845 634 1414 (Adult helpline)
Tel. 0845 634 7650 (Youth helpline)

Enuresis Resource and Information
Centre
34 Old School House
Britannia Road
Kingswood
Bristol BS15 8DB
Tel. 0117 960 3060 (Administration)
Tel. 0117 960 3060 (Helpline)

Foundation for the Study of Infant
Deaths
Artillery House
11–19 Artillery Row
London SW1P 1RT
Tel. 0870 787 0885 (Administration)
Tel. 0870 787 0554 (Helpline)

ISSUE – The National Fertility
Association
114 Lichfield Street
Walsall
West Midlands WS1 1SZ
Tel. 01922 722888

La Leche League (Great Britain)
PO Box 29
West Bridgford
Nottingham NG2 7NP
Tel. 0115 981 5599 (Administration)
Tel. 0845 120 2918 (Helpline)

ME Association
4 Top Angel
Buckingham Industrial Park
Buckingham
Bucks MK18 1TH
Tel. 0870 444 8233 (Administration)
Tel. 0870 444 1835 (Members)
Tel. 0871 222 7824 (Non-members)

Medical Advisory Service for
Travellers Abroad (MASTA)
Moorfield Road
Yeadon
Leeds
West Yorkshire LS19 7BN
Tel. 0113 238 7525 (Administration)
Tel. 01452 331131 (Helpline)

MedicAlert
1 Bridge Wharf
156 Caledonian Road
London N1 9UU
Tel. 020 7833 3034

Mencap
123 Golden Lane
London EC1Y 0RT
Tel. 020 7454 0454

Miscarriage Association
c/o Clayton Hospital
Northgate
Wakefield
West Yorks WF1 3JS
Tel. 01924 200795 (Administration)
Tel. 01924 200799 (Helpline)

National Asthma Campaign
Providence House
Providence Place
London N1 0NT
Tel. 020 7226 2260 (Administration)
Tel. 08457 010203 (Helpline)

National Back Pain Association –
BackCare
16 Elmtree Road
Teddington
Middlesex TW11 8ST
Tel. 020 8977 5474

National Childbirth Trust
Alexandra House
Oldham Terrace
London W3 6NH
Tel. 0870 770 3236 (Administration)
Tel. 0870 444 8707 (Helpline)

National Eczema Society
Hill House
Highgate Hill
London N19 5NA
Tel. 020 7281 3553 (Administration)
Tel. 0870 241 3604 (Helpline)

NSPCC (National Society of the
Prevention of Cruelty to Children)
Weston House
42 Curtain Road
London EC2A 3NH
Tel. 020 7825 2500 (Administration)
Tel. 0808 800 5000 (Helpline)

Parentline Plus
520 Highgate Studios
53–79 Highgate Road
London NW5 1TL
Tel. 020 7284 5500 (Administration)
Tel. 0808 800 2222 (Helpline)
(See telephone directory for regional
helplines)

Psoriasis Association
Milton House
7 Milton Street
Northampton NN2 7JG
Tel: 01604 711129

Relate – National Marriage
Guidance
Herbert Gray College
Little Church Street
Rugby
Warwickshire CV21 3AP
Tel. 01788 573241

Release – The National Drugs and
Legal Helpline
388 Old Street
London EC1V 9LT
Tel. 020 7729 5255

RNIB (Royal National Institute for
the Blind)
105 Judd Street
London WC1H 9NE
Tel. 020 7388 1266 (Administration)
Tel. 08457 669999 (Helpline)

RNID (Royal National Institute for
Deaf People)
19–23 Featherstone Street
London EC1Y 8SL
Tel. 020 7296 8000 (Administration)
Tel. 0808 808 0123 (Helpline)

The Samaritans
The Upper Mill
Kingston Road
Ewel
Surrey KT17 2AF
Tel. 020 8394 8300 (Administration)
Tel. 08457 909090 (National helpline)
(See telephone directory for local
24-hour helplines)

SANDS (Stillbirth and Neonatal
Death Society)
28 Portland Place
London W1B 1LY
Tel. 020 7436 7940 (Administration)
Tel. 020 7436 5881 (Helpline)

Terrence Higgins Trust
52–54 Grays Inn Road
London WC1X 8JU
Tel. 020 7831 0330 (Administration)
Tel. 08451 221200 (Helpline)

Weight Watchers UK
Millennium House
Ludlow Road
Maidenhead
Berkshire SL6 2SL
Tel. 0845 345 1500

Travel

Department of Health
PO Box 777
London SE1 6XH
The DoH provides a number of
leafets, including *Health Advice for
Travellers*, which contains from E111
and details of which countries have
reciprocal arrangements, with the
UK.

Websites
Department of Health:
http://www.dh@gov.uk

Medical Advisory Service for
Travellers Abroad:
http://www.masta.org

Fit for travel: http://www.fit for
travel.scot.nhs.uk

Travel Health UK:
http://www.Travelhealth.co.uk